Penguin Education
Topics in history

9780140800289
AF578212

Alive and well

Medicine and public health
1830 to the present day

Norman Longmate

Norman Longmate read history at Worcester College, Oxford, and later did research at Oxford. He has been a leader writer for the *Evening Standard* and a feature writer for the *Daily Mirror*, and worked for a time in the Education and Training Branch of the Electricity Council. Since 1963 he has been working for the B.B.C., writing and producing history programmes for schools and working in the Secretariat. He has published many books, including five detective stories, but is probably best known for his books on English social history. *King Cholera* (1966) is a history of the cholera epidemics of the nineteenth century, and *The Water Drinkers* (1968) a history of the temperance movement. He is now working on a social history of the Second World War.

Alive and well

Medicine and public health
1830 to the present day

Norman Longmate

Penguin Books

Penguin Books Ltd, Harmondsworth, Middlesex, England
Penguin Books Inc., 7110 Ambassador Road, Baltimore, Md 21207, U.S.A.
Penguin Books Australia Ltd, Ringwood, Victoria, Australia

First published 1970
Copyright © Norman Longmate, 1970

Designed by Arthur Lockwood

Photoset and printed in Malta by
St Paul's Press Ltd
Filmset in Lumitype Century

This book is sold subject to the condition that it shall not, by way of trade or otherwise, be lent, re-sold, hired out, or otherwise circulated without the publisher's prior consent in any form of binding or cover other than that in which it is published and without a similar condition including this condition being imposed on the subsequent purchaser

Contents

1 Health and the towns

A matter of life and death

The aim of medical science is to keep people alive and well — or, if this proves too difficult, at least to keep them alive. The best test of whether the doctors are successful or not over a long period is therefore the individual's average expectation of life. Some people, of course, will be unlucky and will die early, from accident or disease. Some will live an unexpectedly long time — perhaps to a hundred or more. (The oldest Englishman who ever lived, Old Parr, was said to be 152 when he died in 1635.) But in Great Britain today a boy of fifteen can expect on average to live another fifty-five years, till he is seventy, and a girl another sixty years, till she is seventy-five.

Nowadays the average expectation of life does not vary very much between different parts of the country. But 140 years ago, when the subject first began to be seriously studied, there were enormous variations, not merely between different towns but even between different streets. The first report to make this plain was published in 1842. It was written by a civil servant, Edwin Chadwick, of whom more will be heard later.

We find, on inquiry into the sanitary condition of the population of different districts [Chadwick pointed out] that the average chances of life of the people of one class in one street will be 15 years and of another class in a street immediately adjacent, 60 years. In one district of the same town I find . . . the mortality only 1 out of every 57 of the population; and in another district 1 out of every 28 dies annually.

One of Chadwick's tables compared the expectation of life among various classes in the crowded industrial city of Manchester with the thinly populated agricultural county of Rutland.

	Average age of death	
	Manchester	Rutlandshire
Professional persons and gentry, and their families	38	52
Tradesmen and their families (including farmers)	20	41
Mechanics, labourers and their families	17	38

Thus a farm worker in Rutland could expect to live twice as long as a factory worker in Manchester and

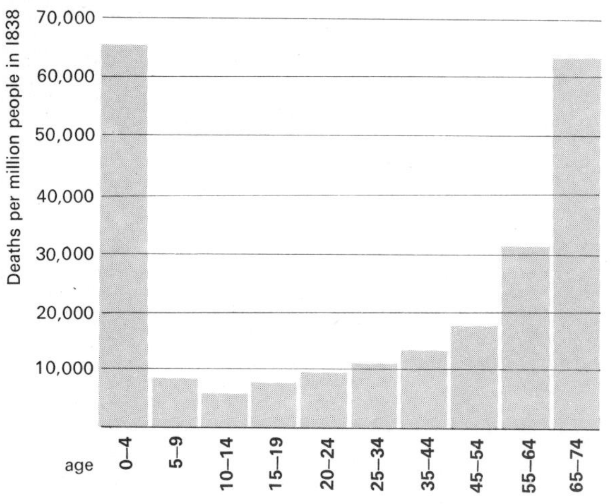

Left This diagram shows how many people died in different age groups during the year 1838. Notice that the table begins with five year periods but later changes to ten years. This has been done to show more accurately the age at which young people died. If all the figures were shown for every ten years, the results would look even more dramatic.

Right An engraving by the French artist Gustave Doré of Wentworth Street, Whitechapel, in about 1870. Doré showed some of the most squalid scenes of London, but in a style full of romantic flourish. Is he right, for example, to show the children so splendidly sad? It is worth noticing the clothes. At this period most of the clothes worn by the poorer people in the towns were old clothes which had once been worn by the middle and upper classes.

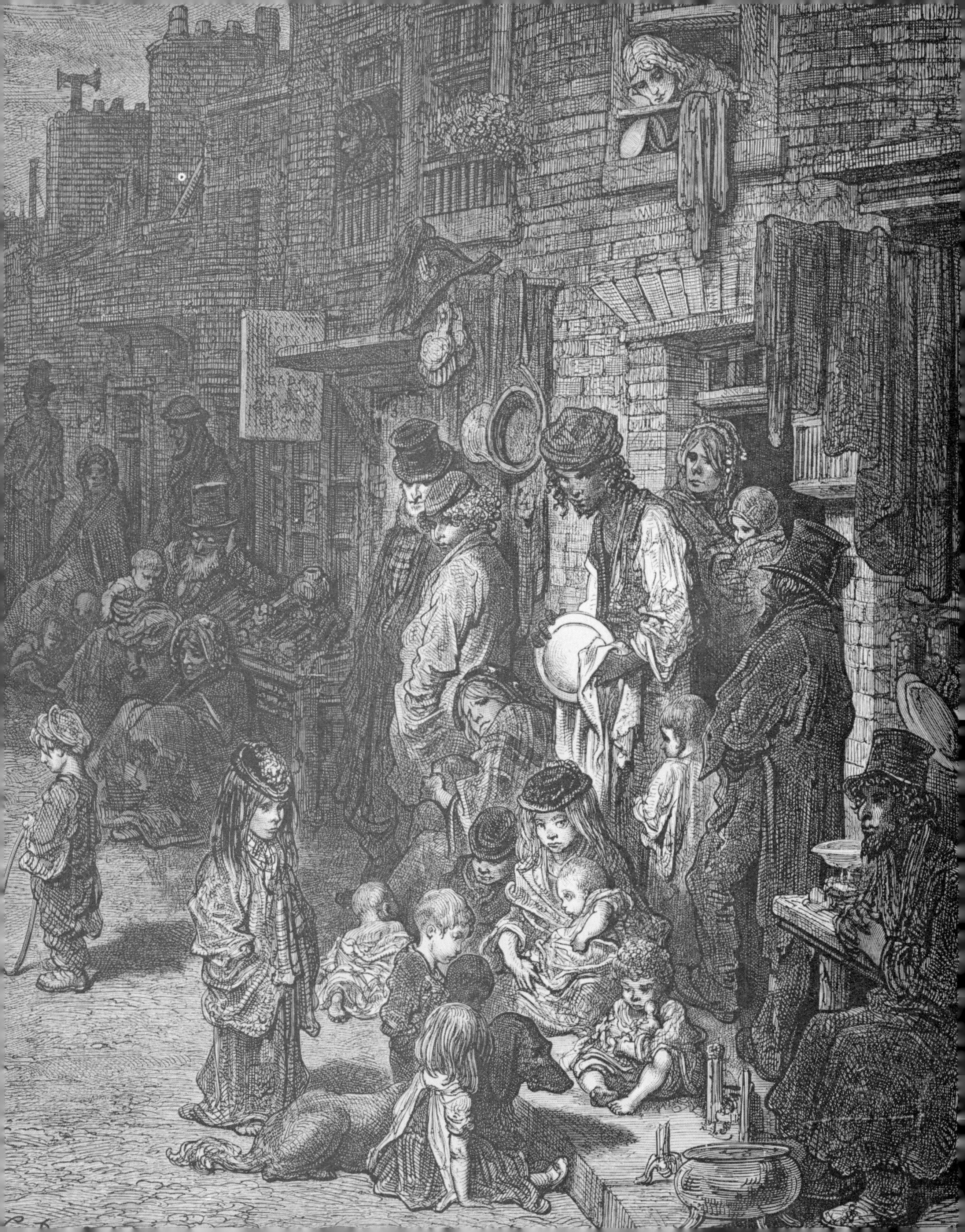

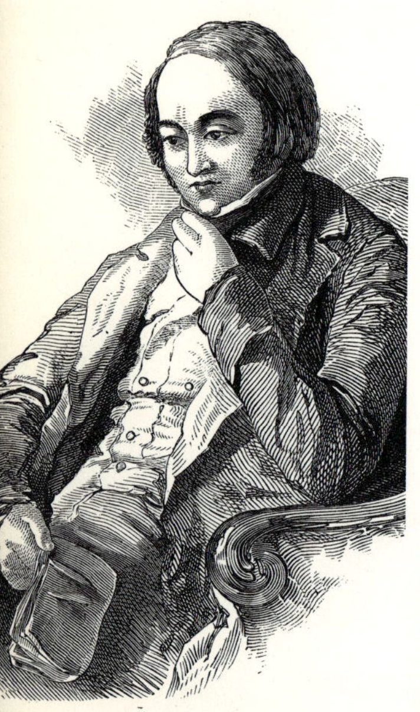

This is the only existing portrait of Chadwick as a young man, at about the time when his *Report* was published. A later picture, which catches more of the character of the man, can be found on page 44.

This table is one of those used by Chadwick to show the chances of life in different places, social classes and in different age groups.

CLASSES.	Total No. of Deaths under 20 Years of Age.	Proportion of Deaths which occurred at the under-mentioned periods of Age.			Proportion of Deaths under 20 Years to Total Deaths.
		Between 0 — 5	Between 5 — 10	Between 10 — 20	
Gentry and Professional Persons, Children of.					
Manchester	21	1 in 3	1 in 24	1 in 54	1 in 3
Leeds	20	1 in 5	1 in 26	1 in 40	1 in 4
Liverpool	61	1 in 3	1 in 11	1 in 23	1 in 2½
Bath	32	1 in 11	1 in 12	1 in 31	1 in 4½
Bethnal Green	33	1 in 5	1 in 20	1 in 13	1 in 3
Strand Union	21	1 in 6	1 in 29	1 in 29	1 in 4
Kendal Union	15	1 in 7	1 in 26	1 in 9	1 in 3
County of Wilts (Unions of) .	25	1 in 9	1 in 40	1 in 13	1 in 5
County of Rutland (Unions of)	4	1 in 4	. .	. .	1 in 7
Total	232	1 in 5	1 in 19	1 in 19	1 in 3½
Farmers, Tradesmen, and Persons similarly circumstanced, Children of.					
Manchester	444	1 in 2	1 in 18	1 in 27	1 in 2
Leeds	425	1 in 2	1 in 18	1 in 18	1 in 2
Liverpool	1,033	1 in 2	1 in 19	1 in 33	1 in 1¾
Bath	78	1 in 4	1 in 24	1 in 30	1 in 3
Bethnal Green	142	1 in 2	1 in 20	1 in 28	1 in 2
Strand Union	99	1 in 3	1 in 20	1 in 25	1 in 2
Kendal Union	47	1 in 4	1 in 35	1 in 14	1 in 3
County of Wilts (Unions of) .	54	1 in 7	1 in 27	1 in 15	1 in 4
County of Rutland (Unions of)	174	1 in 3	1 in 30	1 in 17	1 in 3
Total	2,496	1 in 2¼	1 in 20	1 in 23	1 in 2
Agricultural and other Labourers, Artisans, and Servants, Children of.					
Manchester	3,106	1 in 2	1 in 22	1 in 19	1 in 1½
Leeds	2,245	1 in 2	1 in 14	1 in 14	1 in 1½
Liverpool	4,004	1 in 1½	1 in 15	1 in 33	1 in 1¼
Bath	508	1 in 2	1 in 19	1 in 18	1 in 1¾
Bethnal Green	908	1 in 2	1 in 15	1 in 30	1 in 1½
Strand Union	367	1 in 2	1 in 14	1 in 23	1 in 2
Kendal Union	186	1 in 3	1 in 19	1 in 11	1 in 2
County of Wilts (Unions of) .	954	1 in 3	1 in 21	1 in 14	1 in 2
County of Rutland (Unions of)	293	1 in 3	1 in 18	1 in 18	1 in 2¼
Total	12,571	1 in 2	1 in 17	1 in 20	1 in 1½

even as long as a 'professional person', like a solicitor. A farmer in Rutland could expect to live twice as long as a grocer in Manchester. In fact no one in Manchester, whatever his income or occupation, could expect on average to live to be more than thirty-eight, although Manchester, Chadwick pointed out, was by no means the most unhealthy town in the country.

What caused these great differences? Obviously money had something to do with it, for whether you lived in Manchester or Rutland the better off you were the longer you were likely to live. But money was not the only factor, for the farm worker in Rutland earned, Chadwick discovered, only half as much as the factory worker in Manchester, but still lived more than twice as long. So there were clearly two sets of influences at work, one of which made it healthier to live in the country and the other which increased your chances of life the better off you were, whether you lived in the country or in the town.

Town and country

The most obvious difference between the town dweller and the country dweller was fresh air. The farm labourer's cottage was almost certainly cramped and badly ventilated but he spent his day out of doors and his cottage backed on to fields. Another difference was fresh water—the farm labourer probably had his own well. A third difference was sanitation; he usually had his own lavatory, often an earth closet in a garden shed. Then, although he normally ate less meat than the factory hand because of his low wages, his food often included fresh vegetables and fruit and milk. In other words, the farm labourer enjoyed cleaner air, better water, better sanitation and a better balanced diet than the working man in the town.

In the town

Anyone visiting an industrial city in the 1830s was likely to notice two things at once, the dirt and the

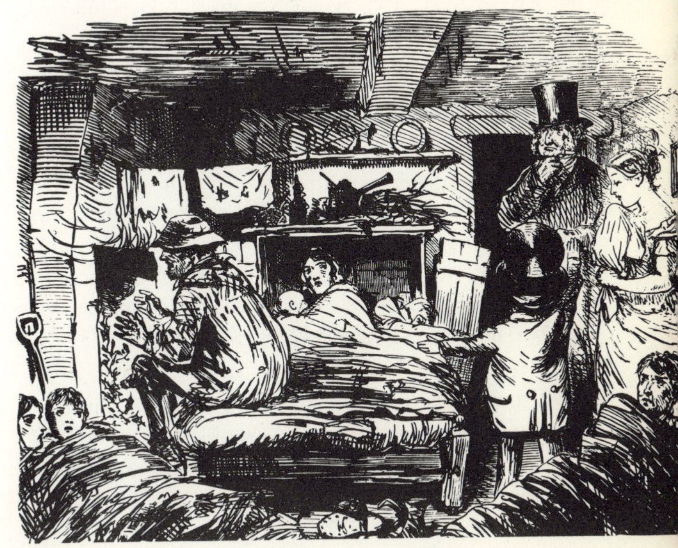

Mr Punch (to Landlord): 'Your stable arrangements are excellent! Suppose you try something of the sort here! Eh?' The standard of living was in general higher in the country, but even so many people were shocked by the condition of country cottages. 'Unless I had seen it,' declared one observer, 'I could not have believed that such a place could exist in England. I had to stoop very low to get inside this habitation of an English agricultural labourer. The total length of this miserable hut was about seven yards, its width three yards, and its height, measured to the extreme point of the thatched roof, about ten feet; the height of the walls, however, not being so much as six feet.' Previously, a man and his wife with six children had lived in this hut, sleeping 'in the "bedroom", nine feet square'.

A photograph of a Glasgow slum tenement building in 1868. No drainpipes: the water is carried away by small runnels, where refuse would also collect.

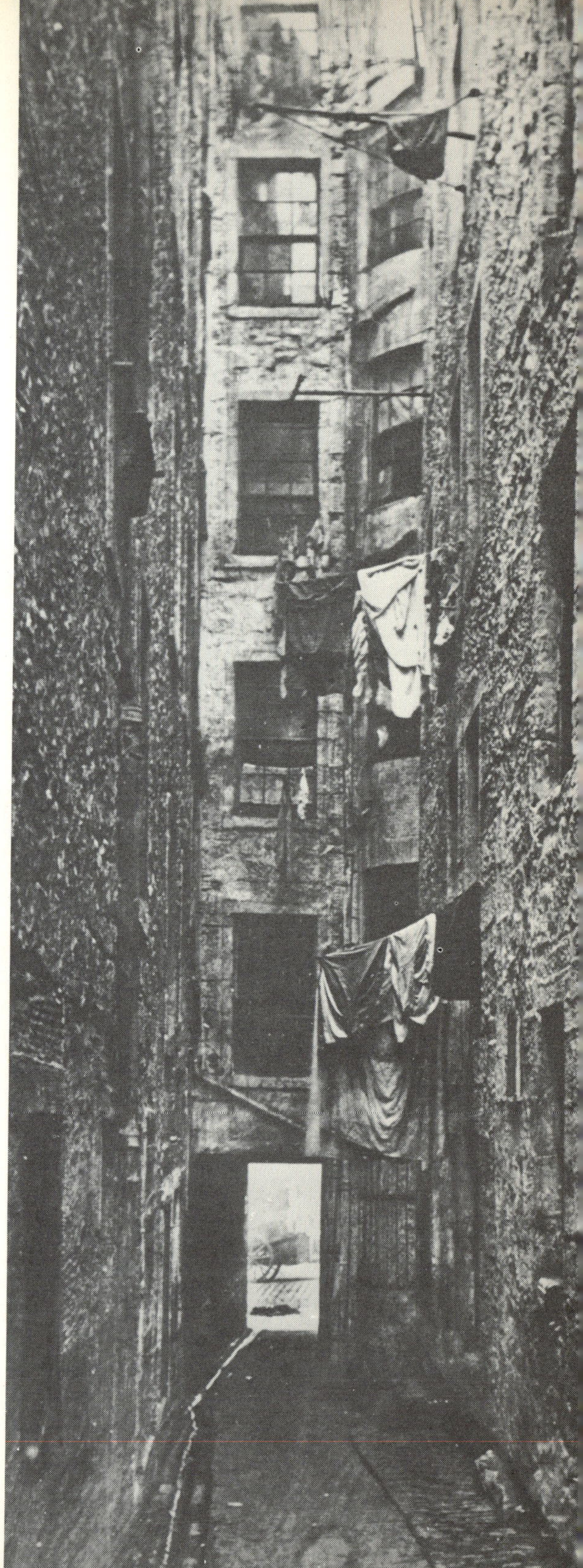

smell. Even the main streets were probably not swept and washed down regularly and in many places there would be potholes in the road and stretches of unpaved footpath. As for the smell, not only was there horse dung everywhere, lying in the road or piled up in the stables behind every large house or shop, but there was very little control over what were called 'nuisances' — firms like tanneries or bone-crushers or slaughter-houses, that poisoned the air for a long way around. This is how a Manchester doctor described one place he visited in 1832:

You descend . . . to the row of houses on the river's edge by interrupted flights of steep steps, and you find yourself when at the bottom in a kind of well or pit, suffocated for want of air (the place admitting of no ventilation) and half poisoned by the effluvia arising from two conveniences which stand in the centre of the well-like area. The brow is covered with filthy refuse — a tripe boiler's works are on one side of the court, a catgut manufactory on the other; in front is the River Irk flowing close under the houses, dyed and defiled by impurities of every kind . . . and on its bank immediately opposite extend large skinneries, with a spacious burial ground . . . behind them.

During the industrial revolution people had poured into the towns to work in the new factories and the population had risen sharply. As there was little public transport, working people had to live close to their work, so houses were squeezed in everywhere. One way of saving space was to build them back to back — there were 2,000 back-to-back houses in Birmingham alone in the 1830s. In Liverpool such places were known as 'blind houses' or 'straight-up houses' and they were often only one room deep. Another doctor described such dwellings as 'the curse of Glasgow'. As the factory workers moved in, the wealthier people often moved further out and houses which had once accommodated only one family were split up to make room for several, just as today large old houses in

Hippolyte Taine, a very intelligent and observant Frenchman, paid three visits to England between 1859 and 1870. The sanitary conditions would have improved since the 1830s, but Taine gives a good impression of what the courts and alleys of a large industrial town must have been like. Over all, Taine found England a place of extreme contrasts: enormous wealth on the one hand, and terrible poverty on the other. This passage is from a modern translation of his *Notes sur l'Angleterre*.

I have seen the lowest quarters of Marseilles, Antwerp and Paris: they come nowhere near this. Squat houses, wretched streets of brick under red roofs crossing each other in all directions and leading dismally down to the river. . . . The grating music from gin cellars can be heard from the street; sometimes the violinist is a negro, and through open windows one sees unmade beds and women dancing. Three times in ten minutes I saw crowds collect round doorways, attracted by fights, especially by fights between women. One of them, her face covered with blood, tears in her eyes, drunk, was trying to fly at a man while the mob watched and laughed. And as if the uproar were a signal, the population of the neighbouring 'lanes' came pouring into the street, children in rags, paupers, street women, as if a human sewer were suddenly clearing itself.

A few of the women show vestiges of former cleanliness, or wear a new dress; but most of them are in dirty, ill-assorted rags. Imagine what a lady's hat can become after having passed for three or four years from one head to another, been dented against walls, bashed in by blows — for that happens frequently. I noticed numerous black eyes, bandaged noses, cut cheeks. These women gesticulate with extraordinary vehemence; but their most horrible attribute is the voice — thin, shrill, cracked, like that of a sick owl.

From the moment you emerge from the tunnel, the whole place is alive with 'street-boys', barefooted, filthy, turning cartwheels for a penny. They swarm on the stairs down to the Thames, more stunted, more livid, more deformed, more repulsive than the street urchins of Paris; the climate, of course, is worse, and the gin murderous. Among them, leaning against the festering walls, or crouched inert on the steps, are men in the most astonishing rags: nobody who has not seen them can conceive what a frock-coat or pair of trousers can carry in layers of filth. They doze and day-dream, their faces earthy, livid, marbled with fine red lines. It was in this quarter that families were discovered whose only bed was a heap of soot; they had been sleeping on it for some months. For the human being reduced to these conditions there is only one refuge: drunkenness.

'Not drink!' said one desperate man, in the course of an inquiry, 'I'd rather die at once.'

A passing tradesman warned me, 'Look out for your pockets, sir.' And a policeman advised me to keep out of certain 'lanes'.

I did, however, walk through several of the widest ones. . . . Other narrow alleys, and dusty yards, were foul with the smell of rotting, old clothes and decorated with rags and linen hung out to dry. There were swarms of children. At one time in a narrow alley, I had fourteen or fifteen all round me, dirty, bare-foot, one tiny girl carrying an infant, a baby still at breast but whose whitish head was completely bald. Nothing could be more dismal than these livid little bodies, the pale, stringy hair, the cheeks of flabby flesh encrusted with old filth. They kept running up, pointing out the 'gentleman' to each other with curious and avid gestures. Their mothers watched from doorways with dull, uninterested eyes. Their interiors were visible, exiguous, sometimes a single room in which the family lives, breathing the foetid air. The houses are generally of a single story, low, dilapidated, kennels to sleep and die in. What can it be like in winter when, during weeks of continuous rain and fog, the windows remain closed? And in order that each numerous brood shall not die of hunger, it is essential that the father abstain from drink, be never out of work and never ill! . . .

The impression is not one of debauchery, but of abject, miserable poverty. One is sickened and wounded by this deplorable procession. . . . Here is a festering sore, the real sore on the body of English society.

Hippolyte Taine

towns are often divided up into flats or bed-sitting-rooms. In the 1830s, however, every room, including the cellars, might house a whole family. Liverpool was particularly notorious for its cellar dwellings. A Liverpool businessman described in a newspaper a tour of one district he made one Sunday morning in 1832.

In all the houses we visited, with a few exceptions . . . each single room from eight to eleven feet square . . . is inhabited by one, sometimes two, families, in which they both eat, drink, cook, wash and sleep. These houses are in general in a dilapidated state, with broken doors, mouldering walls tumbling to ruin, broken windows, in some cases no windows at all, and some without fireplaces; some inhabited the dark, damp cellars so low that you cannot stand upright in them, and not infrequently subject to floods of water; in general these places are filthy in the extreme.

The very worst conditions in most towns were to be found in courts and alleys, narrow passages running off other streets and packed with small houses. Many courts were almost unventilated, since they were entered at one end under a narrow archway and were shut in at the other; some lacked even a name. When doctors in Oxford in 1854 were asked to suggest improvements one recommended 'the naming and legibly posting up of the name of numerous courts and alleys in the poorer districts of the town', because, as he said, the very existence of places without a name was easily forgotten. The 'scavengers' or dustmen who were employed to keep the main streets clean rarely went into the courts, which were usually undrained, so that stepping stones might be provided, as in a country stream, to enable a visitor to cross from one side to the other. In one court in Westminster, only twenty feet wide, all the domestic rubbish, including human excrement, was kept in the houses until the residents could stand it no longer, then thrown into the central space, which became 'a pool of black, stagnant filth'. The atmosphere inside such houses in hot weather was indescribable; even hardened doctors examining patients indoors had to rush outside to be sick or, if attending a confinement, would wait outside in the comparatively fresh air until the actual moment of the birth.

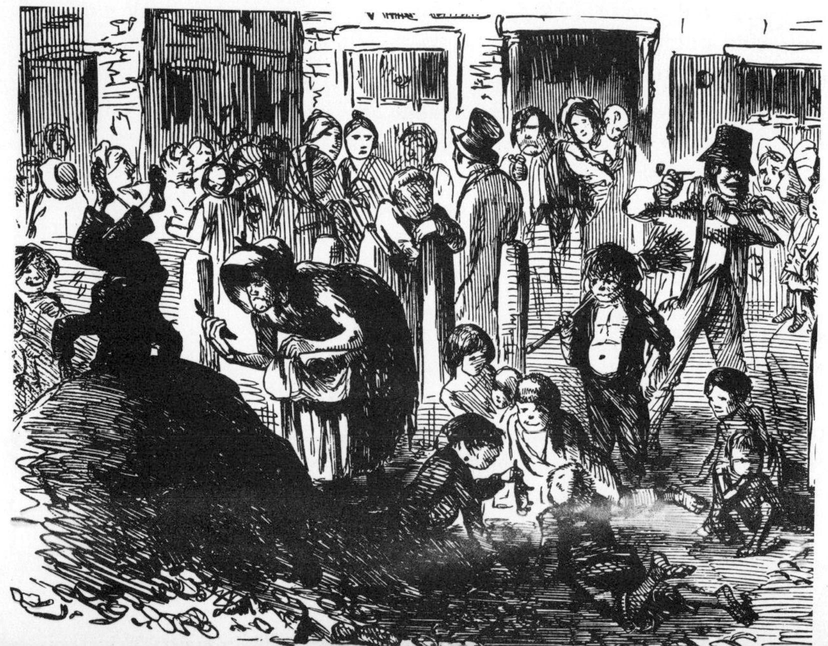

A drawing showing one of London's courts around 1850. Since there were no arrangements for taking away the refuse, this would generally be just thrown out into the courtyard. If it were left for long enough, it was often possible to sell the dungheap to a merchant. Naturally it was usually left — nobody could afford to turn away the prospect of a bit of extra income.

This page from *Sphere* magazine dates from 1875, when people had begun to realize that something had to be done about the towns.

BIRMINGHAM IMPROVEMENTS UNDER THE ARTISANS' AND LABOURERS' DWELLINGS' IMPROVEMENT ACT, 1875

THE present age has been called the age of great cities. For a century past, but still more noticeably during the last thirty years, the chief centres of population have increased immensely in size. This enlargement is, of course, chiefly due to the expansion of trade and enterprise, to locomotive facilities, and to the increase of population which has been stimulated by these improvements. Another cause, which did not exist in less civilised days, conduces to the rapid growth of cities. When war was the rule and peace the exception, every town was virtually more or less a fortress, and, for the sake of protection, people packed their houses closely together within the boundaries of the city walls. Nowadays, every citizen who can afford it tries to have his family abode beyond the reach of the smoke and noise of the central districts, and so a ring of new buildings is added annually to the circumference of the city. One of the most serious evils of modern times results from this tendency to emigrate towards the suburbs. The closely packed houses of the older districts, which were never too healthy, are deserted by the rich and prosperous, and, when in a state of decay and dilapidation, become tenanted by the very poor, who crowd these tenements to an extent never contemplated by those who built them. Intemperance, improvidence, and uncleanliness are confirmed and intensified by the miserable character of these habitations. In nearly every town in the kingdom there may be found what may be styled a mediæval nucleus of this sort; in some instances, as in our own City of London, the old buildings are gradually replaced by structures intended solely for business purposes; but even then one evil is only replaced by another, since the poor, having no dwellings at hand, are compelled to travel long distances to and from their work. For many years philanthropists pondered over the mischief arising from this condition of things, and palliative measures were introduced by individuals and charitable associations; but nothing, as far as we are aware, was accomplished on a comprehensive scale until the passage of a Local Improvement Act in Glasgow, in 1866. That Act has only been taken up extensively during the last five years. Within that time the Corporation have expended upwards of 1,500,000*l.*, have

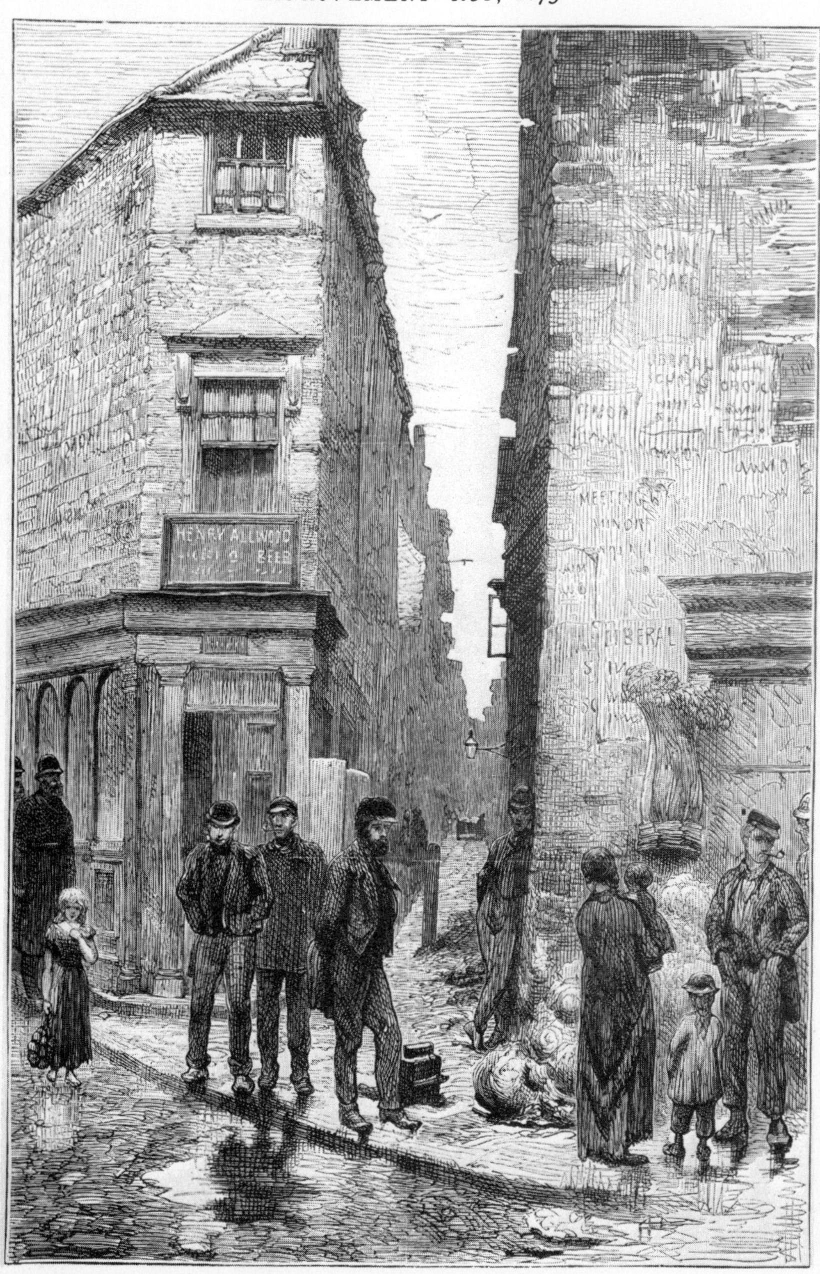

displaced 21,000 persons from unwholesome houses, and have erected within the municipal boundaries healthy dwellings for about 150,000 persons. In 1875 an Act entitled the "Artisans and Labourers' Dwellings Improvement Act" received the assent of Parliament. This Act confers on the sanitary authorities of all towns of more than 25,000 inhabitants very extensive powers of dealing with unwholesome and dilapidated houses, especially as regards compulsory power to buy land or other property, as formerly any owner who chose to be cantankerous or greedy could paralyse any contemplated municipal improvement which touched his property.

Mr. Cross's Act has recently been taken up in good earnest by the authorities of Birmingham—a town which, though exceptionally salubrious among great cities as far as advantages of site are concerned, yet has, in its central districts, a miserable region of damp, dilapidation, and decay; where the deaths are twice as numerous as in the suburb of Edgbaston—young children die especially fast, as one of the tenants pithily put it, "There's more bugs than babies"—where perfect health is unknown and decent habits almost impossible. Those who have read Mr. Councillor White's graphic description of the condition of St. Mary's Ward will not deem the above expressions a whit too strong. A plan of improvement, drawn up in accordance with the representations of the Medical Officer of Health, has been brought forward by Mr. White and carried before the Council, and it is gratifying to add that it was unanimously accepted, although a few aldermen and councillors abstained from voting owing to motives of delicacy, because they owned property on the line of intended demolition. It will be perceived, on reference to our map, that the proposed scheme is one of an extensive character; it is intended to combine the advantage of new and improved dwellings for the poorer classes with convenient thoroughfares. Those who know Birmingham are aware how much a route for vehicular traffic is needed between New Street and Bull Street. In the proposed improvements a new thoroughfare will commence in New Street, opposite the Exchange, and will be carried right through, across Legge Street and Bagot Street, into the Aston Road. New subsidiary side streets will also be made, and the

Clean water and fresh

In most towns in the 1830s clean water was even scarcer than fresh air. Only comfortably off families had a supply piped into their own homes, and even this would be turned on only for a few hours a day. In an early Victorian house the news that the water was running would cause general excitement, as the maids hurried to fill every possible receptacle before the tap ran dry; even the mistress of the house might lend a hand. People without their own supply relied on butts which collected rain water, on wells, often contaminated by water draining into them from the street, and on public taps or standpipes serving a whole street or estate. These would usually only be on for an hour a day during the week and were turned off from midday on Saturday until Monday morning. Long before the water was due to come on a queue would form of people carrying buckets and saucepans and as the time approached for it to be turned off men and women might fight to get to the front. Water selling was a profitable business. Water sellers would tour the streets with a horse-drawn cart carrying a huge cask and offering water at a halfpenny a bucket, or on foot with two huge buckets suspended on a frame across their shoulders, shouting 'Clean water and fresh!' Once obtained, water was stored in the kitchen in open buckets —one doctor at this period described seeing some covered 'with a black scum'. In Exeter, in 1832, when the local waterworks owner agreed to supply water to clean the streets he made it a condition that there should be no 'dipping' by people scooping free water out of the gutters as it ran past their door. In Birmingham as late as the 1870s the Water Company's piped service ran only three days a week and was available to only half the population; the rest used surface wells, often filthy, and water carts. Water-stealing was a common crime. The famous reforming mayor of Birmingham, Joseph Chamberlain, remarked that many magistrates had told him that:

> of all their duties the saddest is that of registering convictions against poor people . . . for stealing that which is one of the first necessities of life. They might almost as well be convicted of stealing air.

Another famous reformer, Dr Southwood Smith of London, agreed. 'It is,' he said, 'fortunate that air is more accessible than water and that its supply does not depend on landlords and water companies.' In one estate of 200 houses in Whitechapel, East London, there was not a single pump, 'the inhabitants', a local

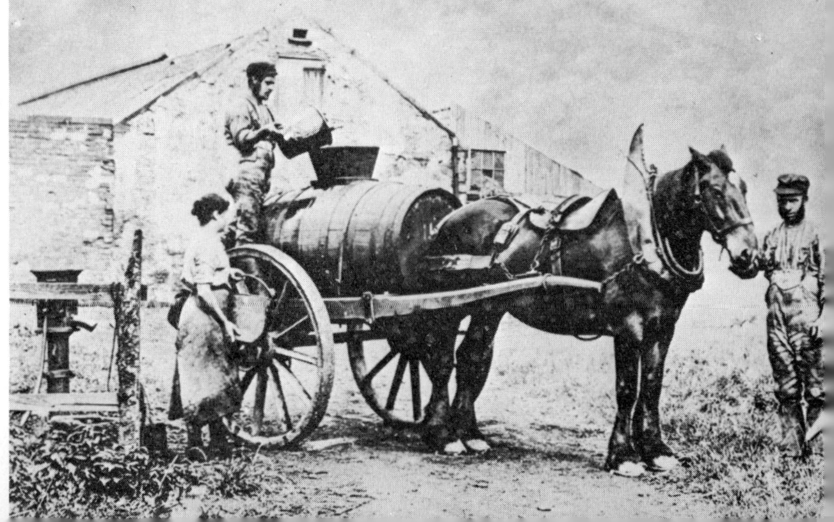

A water cart photographed in 1887. Piped water was regarded as a great luxury, and most people obtained theirs from a cart like this or from a street pump, although the pumps were often turned off for most of the day. Some people even scooped water straight from the nearest river.

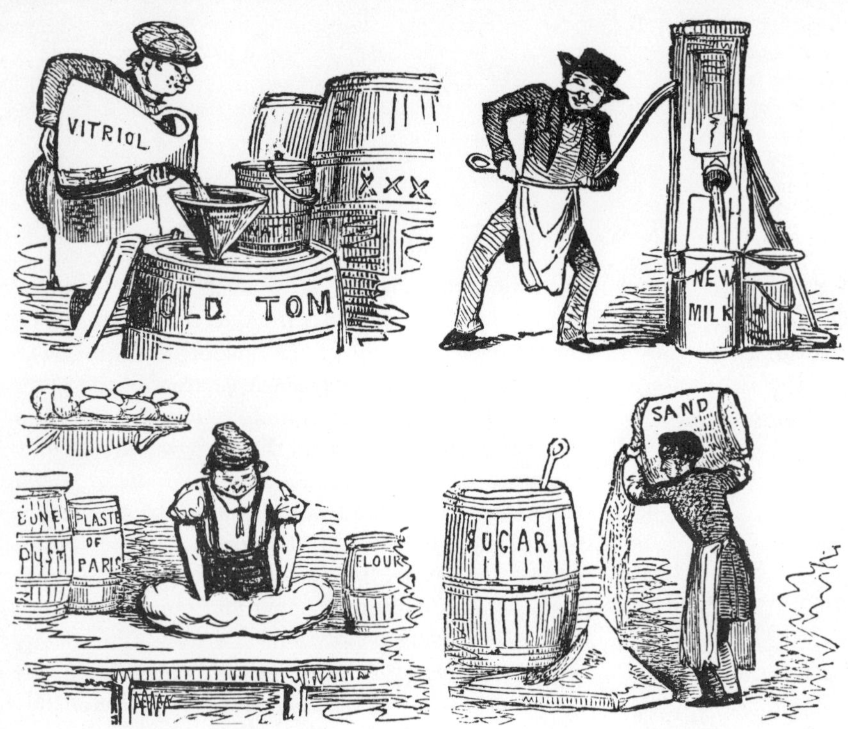

A comment on the purity of food. Magazines of the time frequently contained advice to housewives on how to test the foods they bought. Even these would not have helped very much, however, since the tradesmen were often extremely ingenious and inventive about their faking. There was a brisk trade amongst serving women, for example, in used tea leaves.

official reported, 'having to go to a distant pump or beg of their neighbours, who have had it laid on at their own expense and who for giving it are liable to punishment.' When public pumps were provided there were never enough of them. A part of St Pancras, in central London, in which 170,000 people lived, had only thirteen pumps between them, one to every 13,000 people. In Rotherhithe, until 1843, there was no public supply at all, and people dipped buckets in the River Thames to supply their needs.

Water obtained in this way was, however, often undrinkable, especially if there happened to be a chemical works or factory, or the outlet from a sewer, nearby. One tributary of the River Thames in London was nicknamed 'the Stinking Ditch' and in 1853 a special Commission of Enquiry investigating the water supply in Newcastle, which was drawn from the River Tyne, reported that it 'is variously described as "bad", "very bad" . . . or "shockingly bad"'.

It was not surprising that, until well on into the nineteenth century, few working people drank much water. The everyday drink was beer, which cost only twopence a pint. Apart from the very poor, who were permanently half-starved, the average family did not eat badly: bread, potatoes, meat, fish, cheese — all were reasonably cheap. The importance of a balanced diet was not understood, however; a doctor was more likely to prescribe wine for an ailing child than milk or fresh fruit, which were luxuries. Some food, too, was adulterated with cheaper substances by the grocer to increase his profit. 'If your "strong tea" tastes of ink, examine it with a magnet, to see if it contains iron, added to cheat you in the weight,' advised one doctor's *Manual of Diet*. 'Sugar — the baser sort — always contains dirt, sand and mites . . . . Grocers get from handling it "grocers itch".' There were many complaints, too, about chemicals being added to the poor man's beer — either salt to make him more thirsty or tobacco to make it seem stronger. An experienced beer drinker wrote in 1824 that 'it has seldom been my fortune, in a great number of years, to taste unadulterated purchased ale', while government inspectors between 1844 and 1856 found that 142 of 215 samples of beer they tested were adulterated.

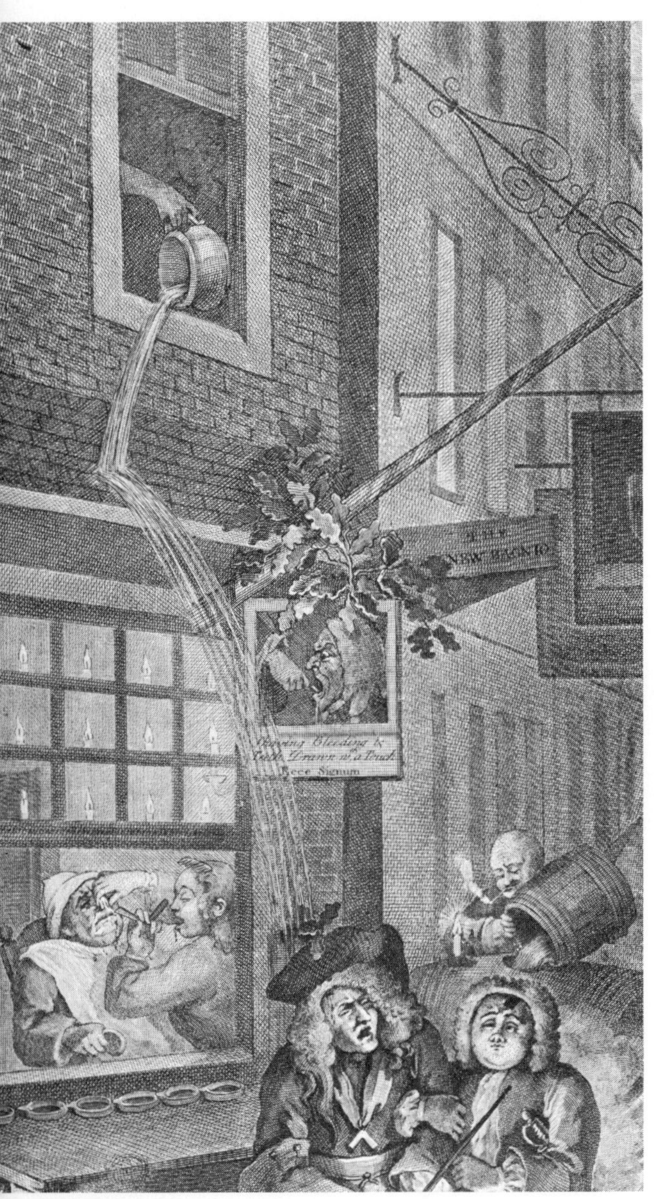

In Scotland anyone hearing the cry 'Gardy loo!' — Scots for 'Gardez l'eau!' — was advised to look about him smartly. It meant that someone was about to empty the contents of a chamber pot or washing bowl out of the window. The call is sometimes said to be the origin of the modern slang word for a lavatory. The ground floor of this house is a barber's shop, though the barber himself is a bit the worse for drink. The sign reads 'Shaving, Bleeding and Teeth Drawn with a Touch'.

The privy problem

But by far the greatest threat to the health of the town dweller for most of the nineteenth century was the lack of proper sanitation. A lavatory of their own was for a working-class family a luxury, and even in a middle-class household the privy would probably be squeezed into a small, unventilated cupboard, would be flushed rarely, and would drain into an outdoor cesspit liable to overflow. The older parts of a town might have sewers but they did not cover the newly built terraces, run up cheaply and quickly to house the rapidly rising population, and were often in any case unsatisfactory. Since there was no other means of cleaning them out regularly, sewers were commonly built of brick and made large enough to allow a man to walk through them, so that dirt accumulated in the corners and cracks, and they usually drained into any convenient river. Normally in a poor district all the families in a house, or row of houses, would share one outdoor privy, which was rarely emptied or cleaned. Some landlords made no provision for sanitation at all and families had to rely on chamber-pots, which were emptied on the nearest piece of waste ground or in the street. In one part of Leeds, in 1839, it was discovered that 'the streets had become so full of ashes, filth and refuse of every description that their surfaces were far above their original level'. The Leeds Corporation admitted that 'the greater part of the town is in a most filthy condition'. Of the 586 streets in the town, 231 were classified as 'bad' or 'very bad' and some were actually impassable for the rubbish heaped up in them. Much of this rubbish consisted of human excrement. In three adjoining streets, containing 452 persons, there were only two conveniences, neither of them fit for use. In Boot and Shoe Yard, with 340 people, there were only three privies, one of which — not surprisingly, perhaps, since the nearest water was a quarter of a mile away — had not been cleaned for seven years. When the dirt was at last cleared away from them it filled seventy cart-loads.

Nor was Leeds unique. In Clayton's Yard, North Shields, sixty loads of manure were removed from one dung heap, and others were found in yards and even in empty rooms inside houses. In Duke Street, Tynemouth, only five families out of 196 had a privy; the rest had to manage as best they could. In Sunderland a doctor in 1832 described the 'narrow passages, crowded with the thickly populated houses of the poor, badly paved, with a gutter in the centre, where all the filth of human habitations is needlessly thrown'. Prudent people, however, took more care of it; in some streets there were trap doors leading into cellars, where sewage was dumped until it could be collected and sold as manure.

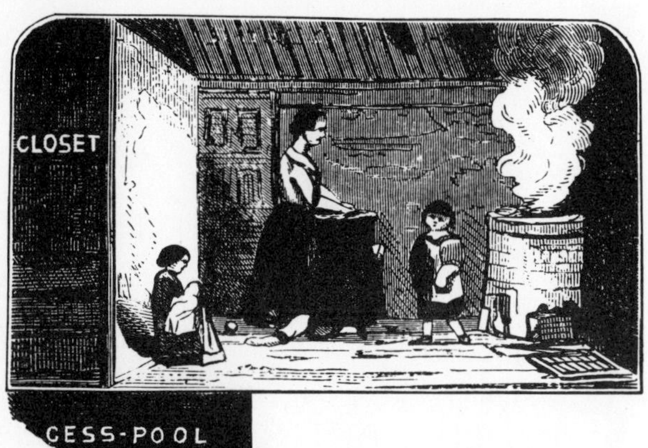

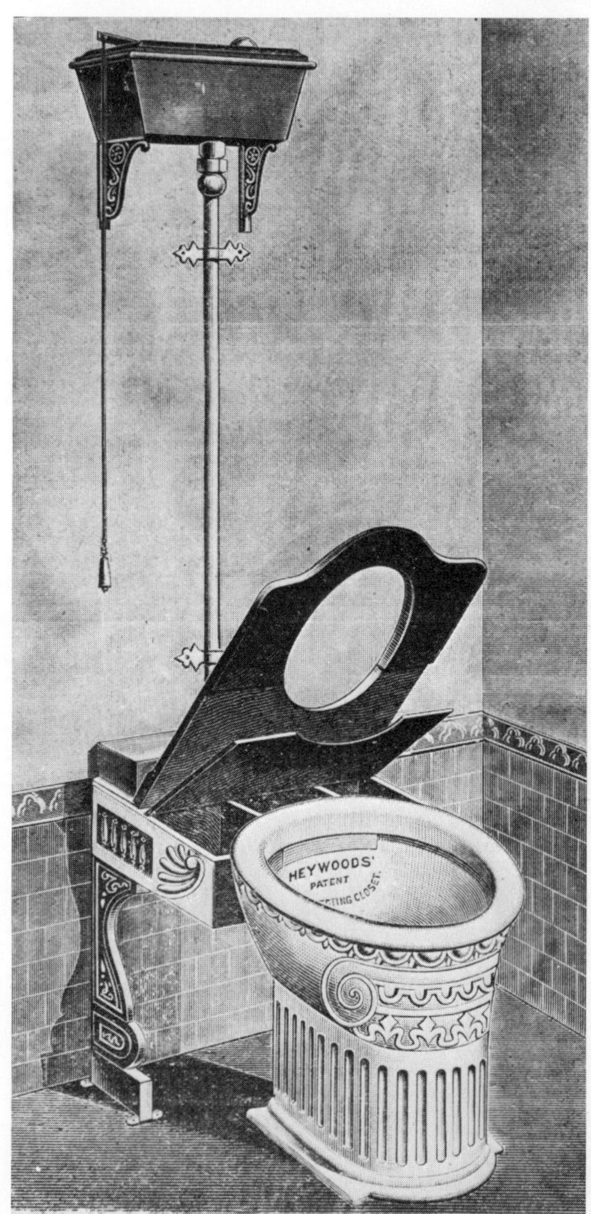

This diagram shows a cesspool directly under the washroom of a London house. On the right is an early version of a water closet — this one was offered for sale in 1889. But even when the new machine had been installed there was still the problem of where the waste could be piped to.

Similar conditions existed throughout the British Isles and improvement was slow in coming. A government commission of inquiry described Merthyr Tydfil in South Wales, in 1844, as being 'in a sad state of neglect . . . . Some parts of the town are complete networks of filth . . . . During the rapid increase of this town no attention seems to have been paid to drainage.' 'In some localities,' reported a local resident, 'a privy was found common . . . to 100 persons or more.' The worst part of the town, containing 1,500 people, was described as 'a labyrinth of miserable tenements and filth'. Even in a small Devonshire village in 1849 a visiting doctor noted that there were few privies; the local residents simply threw their refuse in the sea. As late as 1850 there were still 250,000 cesspools in London; Birmingham was spending £5,000 a year on emptying the buckets of privies; and in Manchester fewer than one house in twenty yet had a water-closet.

Fresh water, too, was still a rarity. The humorous magazine *Punch* said of the 1851 Great Exhibition:

> The contractor is bound to supply, gratis, pure water in glasses to all visitors demanding it; but the Committee must have forgotten that, whoever can produce in London a glass of water fit to drink will contribute the rarest and most universally useful article in the whole exhibition.

Curiously enough, this did not prevent English people looking down on 'dirty foreigners'. A letter in *The Times* urged the need for more 'temporary conveniences' during the Exhibition as 'foreigners are not particular when certain calls of nature press, where they stop to relieve themselves,' and *Punch*, in the same year, carried the cartoon reproduced on this page.

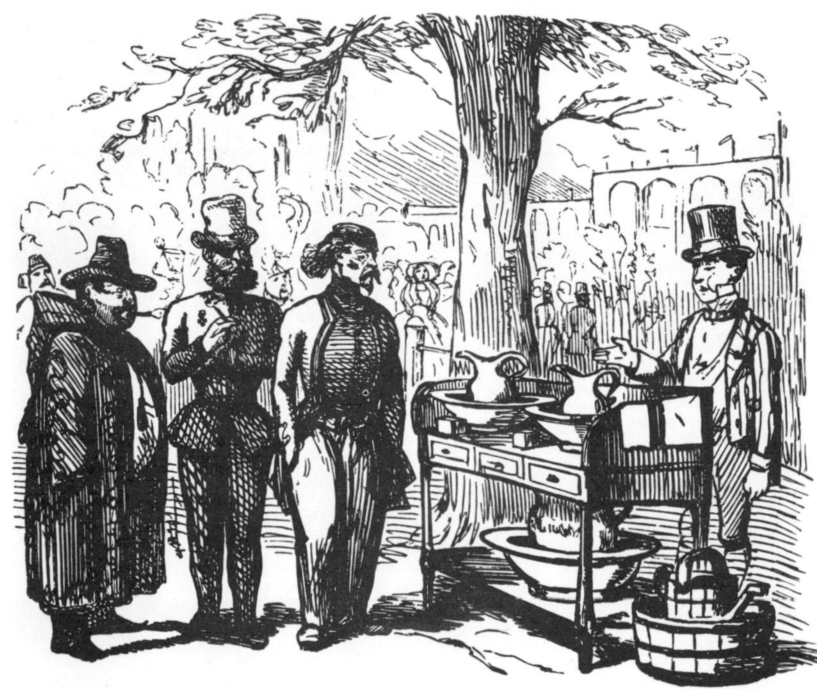

In this *Punch* cartoon, three Frenchmen regard a washbasin. 'Mon Dieu, Alphonse! Look! What do you call that machine there?' In many European countries, hypocrisy came to be known as 'The English Vice'.

Punch in fine rollicking form on 'The Wonders of a London Water Drop'. 'And wondrous indeed is the sense disclosed within the sphere of a little drop of water – of that water which Londoners drink, swallowing daily, myriads and myriads of worlds, whole universes instinct with life, or life in death! . . . Creatures – who shall name them? things in human shape – in all appearance London citizens – aldermen, deputies, common councilmen – are seen disporting in the liquid as in their native element. Behold them, fiercely hustling each other in competition for atomic garbage.'

Small wonder that most working men preferred beer or gin. Drink was one of the major social problems of nineteenth-century England. In the early part of the nineteenth century many families spent a third of their income on alcohol.

THE FOUNTAIN.
SPIRIT
STORE.
FINE
CORDIAL
GIN
DOUBLE
WHISKY

THE FIRST PUBLIC FOUNTAIN ERECTED BY THE
DRINKING FOUNTAIN ASSOCIATION.

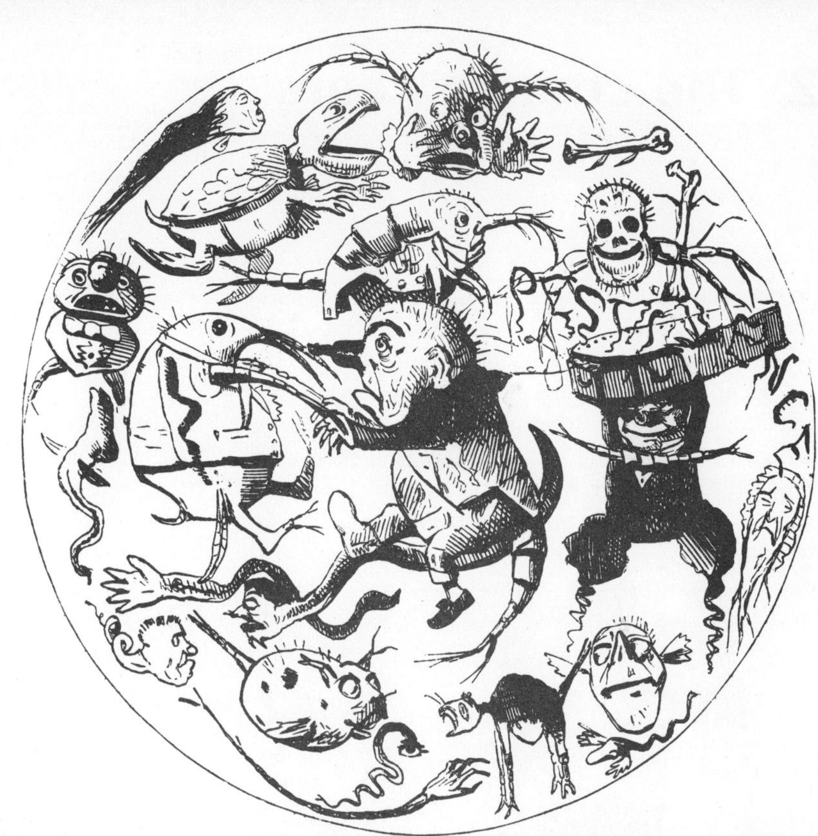

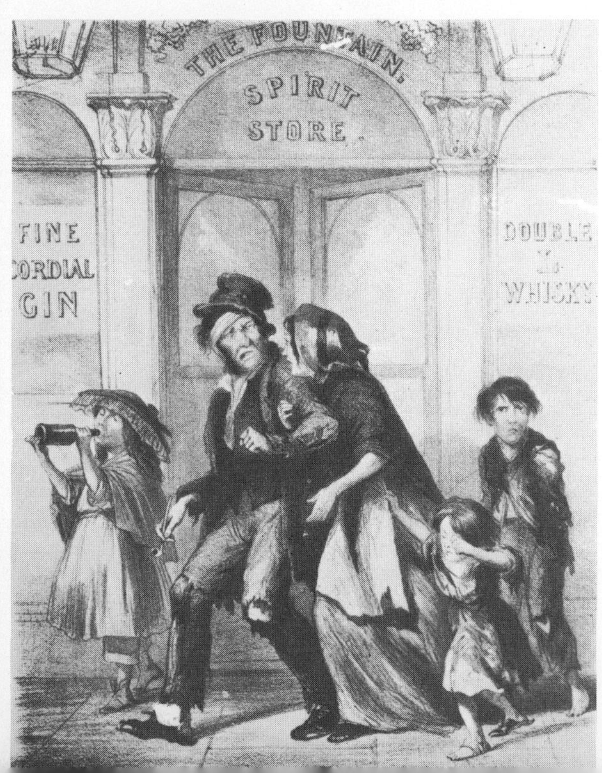

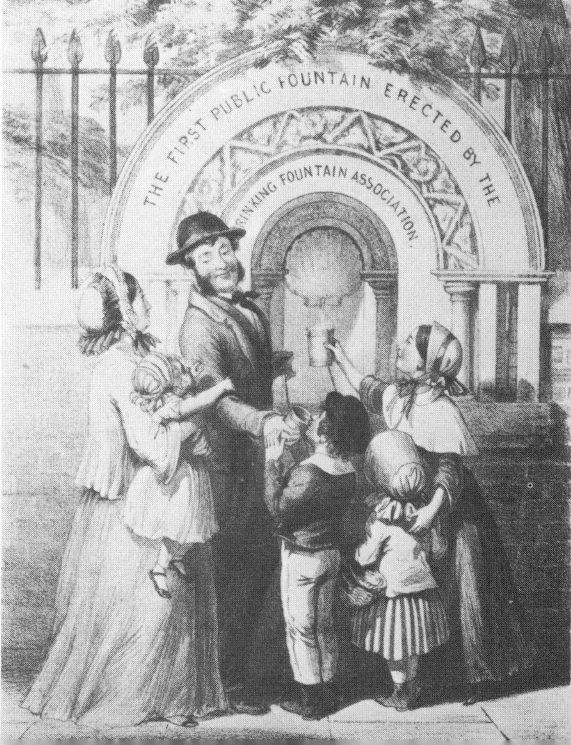

2 The cholera years

No one who had ever walked through the poorer parts of a large city could fail to be aware at this time of the squalor amid which many people lived, but it was the sudden appearance in England of a new disease which first brought the condition of the towns home to the nation as a whole and set in motion what was called 'the sanitary movement' — a campaign for better housing, a purer water supply, cleaner streets, decent drainage, and even for more open spaces and parks and more opportunities for education. News had first reached England in 1818 of a terrible epidemic which was ravaging India. No one had known anything like it before, but as it seemed closest to a form of stomach upset known as 'cholera', and since it came from the East, it became known as the 'Asiatic cholera' or 'Indian cholera'. Those who had seen it at work, however, had other names for it, like 'cholera asphyxia' because it seemed to choke its victims to death, 'the black illness' because their skin and finger nails turned black, and, for obvious reasons, 'the blue vomit'.

Gradually the new disease crept closer to the British Isles, causing panic and thousands of deaths wherever

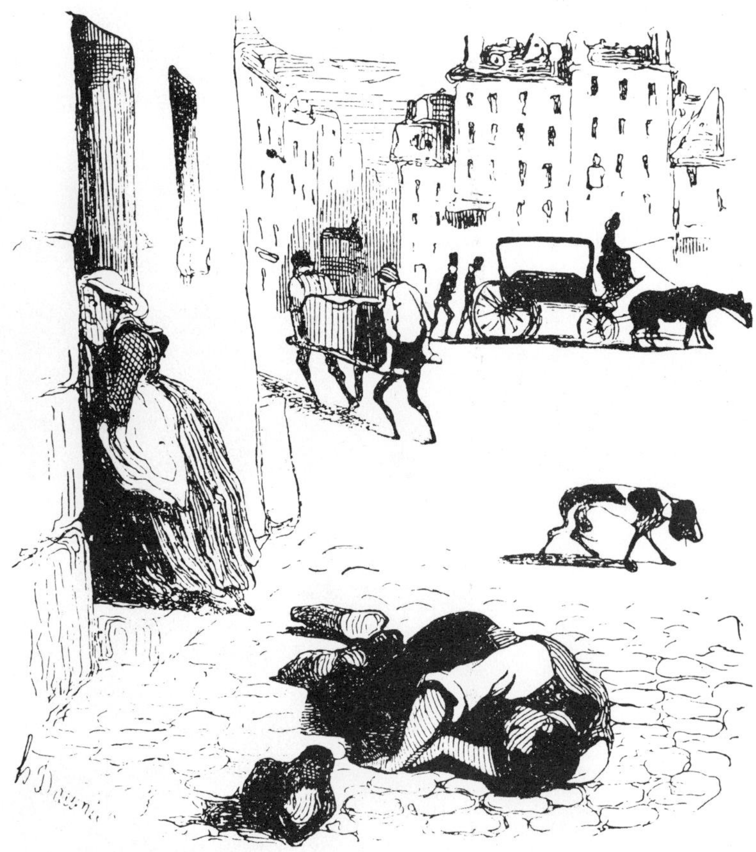

A cholera victim, by the French artist Honoré Daumier.

Right The first news of the Asiatic cholera came from near Calcutta in 1818. A second wave began in 1826. By 1830 the new disease was in Moscow.

it appeared, in Russia, in the Middle East, in the Balkans, and finally in Germany. Although attempts to keep it out of other countries had all failed, the government hoped to prevent cholera from entering the British Isles. Strict measures were introduced: warships patrolled the coast and forced any vessels from infected places to go into special quarantine stations, and in November 1831 an official prayer was issued, for at this time many people thought that epidemics were God's punishment for people's sins:

We acknowledge it to be of Thy goodness alone [ran the prayer] that whilst Thou has visited other nations with pestilence, Thou has so long spared us .... O merciful Father, suffer not thy destroying angel to lift up his hand against us, but keep us as Thou has heretofore done in health and safety.

Another prayer, which a rector in the Midlands issued to his parishioners, hinted that Britain *ought* to be privileged. 'Spare we beseech Thee,' it ran, 'this Thy favoured land.' Epidemics were something that happened to foreigners, not to Englishmen.

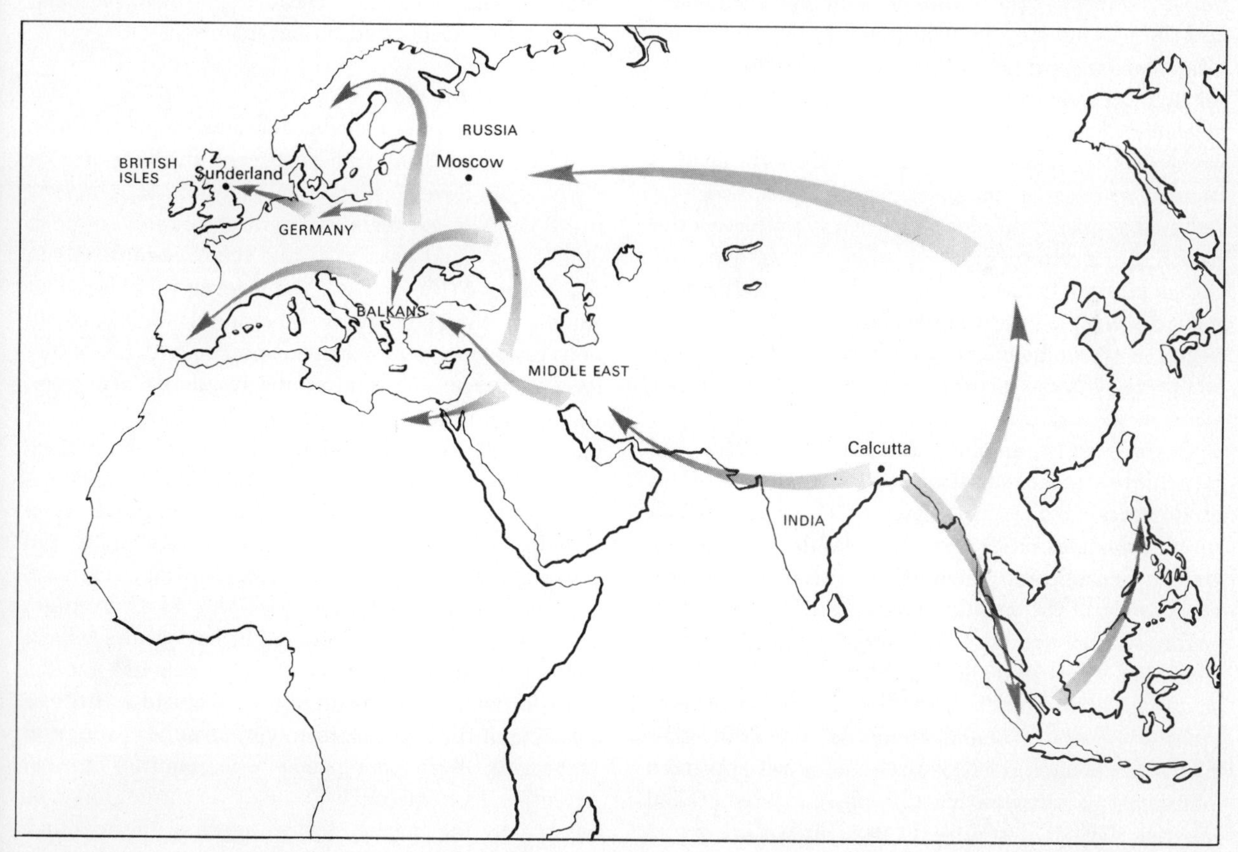

The port of Sunderland in the early nineteenth century, the scene of the entry of cholera into the British Isles.

Local government before 1835

The government was meanwhile taking some more practical steps to prepare for cholera. There was no government department in charge of health so in June 1831 a special, temporary Board of Health was set up, consisting mainly of leading doctors, whose job was to draw up regulations for keeping cholera out and for preventing it spreading if it arrived. In October this central Board advised the setting up in every town and village of 'a local Board of Health, to consist of the chief . . . magistrates, the clergymen of the parish, two or more physicians or medical practitioners, and three or more of the principal inhabitants'. Each local board was supposed to make its own preparations for fighting an epidemic, like earmarking some houses as cholera hospitals, and recruiting unemployed local women as nurses. These local boards were needed because at this time the government did not recognize any real responsibility for permanently protecting the health of the ordinary citizen, which he was expected to look after for himself. When, as in 1831, the government did want to intervene, because an epidemic which began in the slums might easily spread to the districts where 'respectable' people lived, there was no proper system of local government which they could use.

In the country, anything that got done at all would be achieved by the magistrates, who were usually local landowners, farmers or clergymen. The way in which most towns and cities were run at this time was extremely complicated. In many of the older towns a corporation of the wealthy inhabitants was in charge, perhaps appointed for life, and often giving key jobs like that of Inspector of Nuisances, equivalent to a modern Public Health Inspector, to friends or relations who had no qualifications for them. In other places power often belonged to elected or self-appointed committees of the wealthiest people in a parish, called vestries. The real trouble in most urban areas was not that there were too few authorities but too many. Commissioners of Improvements, Commissioners of Sewers, paving boards and lighting boards – all might be responsible for one small part of the job of keeping a town fit to live in, or even for a few yards of one street. Lambeth, in South London, for example, had nine separate boards for keeping the streets lit. Seven different paving boards shared the job of keeping the three-quarters of a mile of the Strand in London in repair, while, a few minutes walk away, in St Pancras, responsibility was divided between sixteen different paving boards – because of which, perhaps, most of the streets had no pavements at all.

The care of the sick

The system of public medical care was equally primitive. The idea that free treatment in illness was a *right* would have seemed startling to almost everyone in 1832. You got medical attention, as you got food, only if you could pay for it, and the local authority in the shape of 'the parish', the leading inhabitants of the district working through their paid officials, would only intervene to stop someone actually dying of disease or starvation – and not always then. There were, by the standards of the time, some fine, long-established hospitals, both in London and in the chief provincial cities, but they were run strictly as a charity and it was not easy to gain admission to them. Often one required a 'letter of recommendation' from some influential person, such as a governor, or one's local clergyman, and though people who were absolutely destitute might be treated in the workhouse infirmaries, these were really intended for inmates of the workhouse and the main consideration in them was to spend as little as possible of the ratepayers' money on either comfort or treatment. Very poor people who required medical attention at home might, though very grudgingly, be treated by the 'parish doctor', often an ill-qualified,

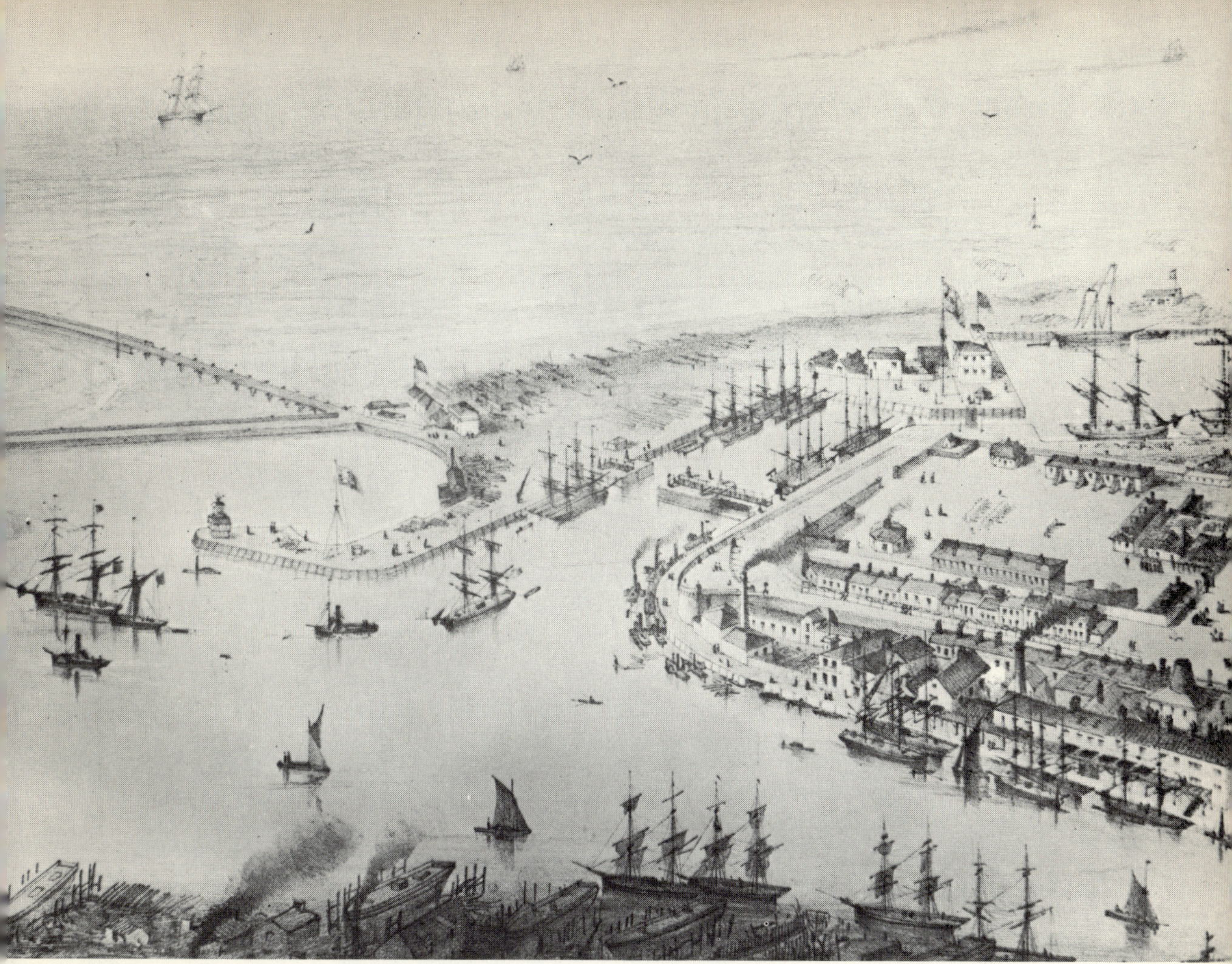

ill-paid young man who barely managed to make a living. Those slightly better off might subscribe to a friendly society (which was sometimes also a thinly disguised trade union) paying a shilling or so a week in return for the services of the society's doctor when they needed him, for sick pay when they could not work and a funeral grant for their relatives if they died. Most people, however, did not belong to a friendly society and it was upon them — the very poorest, and hence the worst fed and worst housed—that the cholera was to fall hardest.

The coming of cholera

The government's efforts to keep cholera out of the British Isles with prayer, quarantine and whitewash, distributed free by local boards of health in a desperate, last minute effort to clean up the cities, failed, and in October 1831 the first case was diagnosed in Sunderland, County Durham, then a flourishing port of about 19,000 people, nearly all working class. They lived mainly in small houses crowded together in narrow lanes or in larger, older houses, split up into tenements; water supply and sanitation were as bad as anywhere and much rubbish and sewage was dumped on the Town Moor, an open space which became one of the centres of the epidemic.

Exactly how the disease was first introduced into the British Isles is still a mystery, but it was probably by a German seaman who managed to evade the quarantine. The first officially recognized case was diagnosed

This gruesome sketch of one of the first victims of the cholera in the British Isles must have been taken from the life.

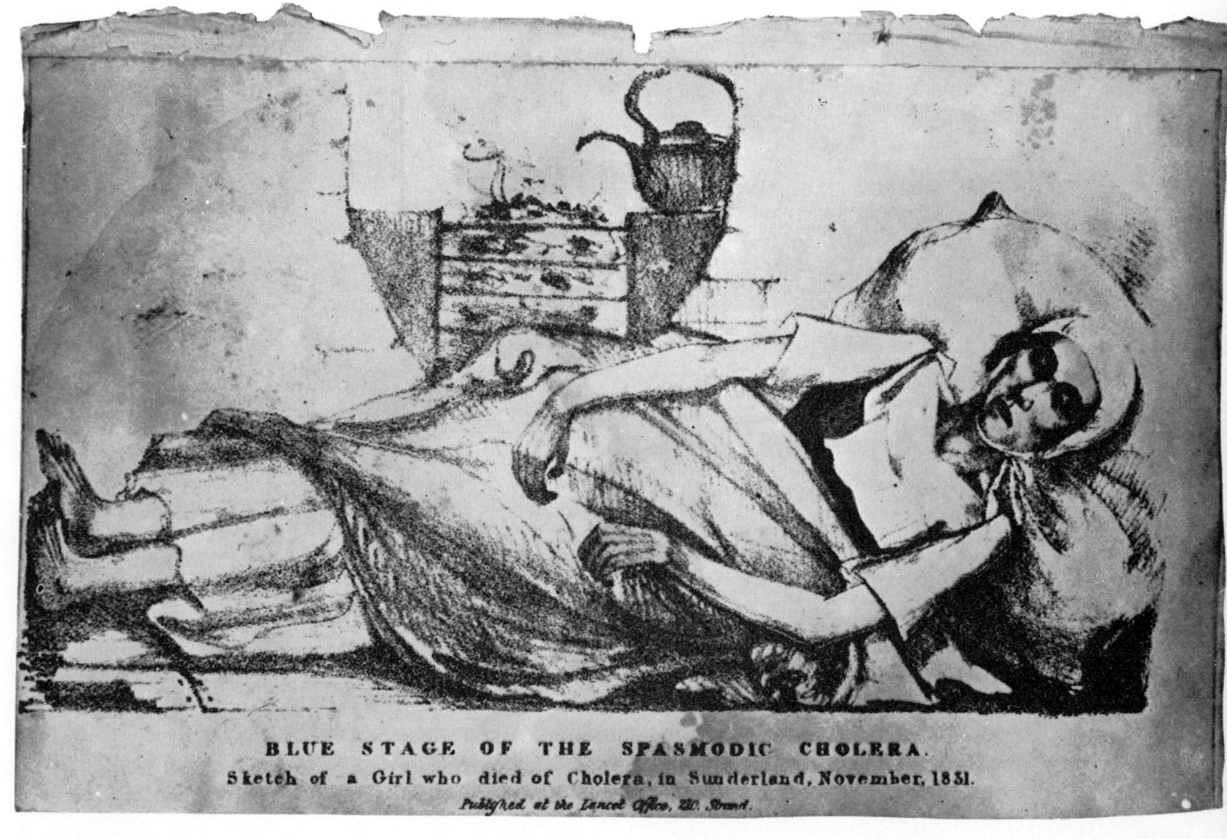

on Sunday afternoon, 23 October 1831. The doctors did their best for the patient, but 'on Wednesday morning, October the 26th,' recorded one, 'he was much weaker, the pulse scarcely beating under the fingers, countenance quite shrunk, eyes sunk, lips dark blue, as well as the skin of the lower extremities; the nails were livid . . . . At 12 o'clock he died.'

Several other cases followed a few days later; by the following weekend the first victim's son was desperately ill, throwing himself about in bed, moaning and biting the bedclothes. Soon after he had died an old woman who had nursed him went to bed in a state of terror. At one a.m. next morning she was awoken by the dreaded symptoms of cholera; by dusk that evening she was dead. Other cases followed, all over the town, but at first the leading local businessmen tried to hush up the existence of cholera in Sunderland, as they were afraid that it would be bad for their trade. They even managed to force most of the local doctors to pretend that they had made a mistake and the disease was not cholera at all. Today, as will be explained later, such a question would be settled beyond argument by bac-

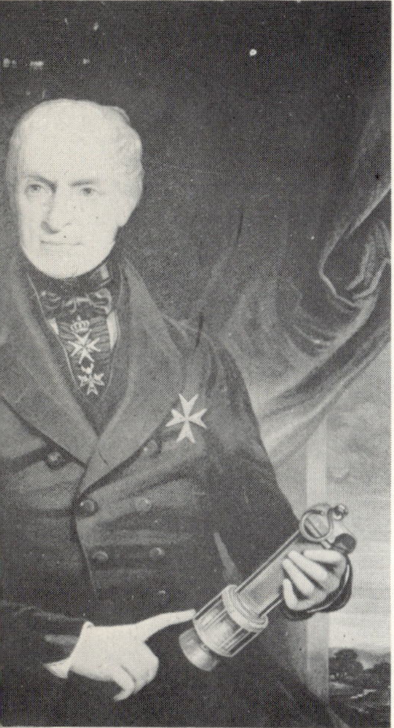

The local Board of Health in Sunderland chose Dr Reid Clanny to head a special committee of doctors. Clanny was an intelligent physician, but knew no more than anyone else about this strange new disease: he was greatly interested, for example, in the possible effects of weather and the atmosphere on the illness. The poster on the right was issued by Clanny to dispel the numerous conflicting rumours about the outbreak of cholera.

CHOLERA MORBUS.

TO THE PUBLIC.

IN justice to the Community, and also to myself, I find it needful to publish the following Facts, which I dare any Man, or set of Men to disprove.

When the Board of Health of this Town was first established, I was called to the Chair of the Medical Department, and many salutary Plans and Regulations were from time to time discussed at our Medical Meetings.

On Tuesday the 1st. of November, at a General Meeting of the Medical Department of the Board of Health, at which all the Members of the Board were invited, I understand the following Medical Gentlemen were present. I give them as far as I am able, according to Seniority; Doctors Clanny, Miller, Atkinson, Brown, Haslewood, Burn, Happer, Ogden, and Croudace—Surgeons, Happer, Croudace, Fothergill, Dixon, Smithson, Holmes, Torbock, Embleton, Cooke, Penman, Mordey, and Maling. Five Cases of Cholera were reported, of which, Four had died in a few days, and the Fifth being at the Point of Death. The following Query was put from the Chair, without comment.

Is it the Opinion of the Medical Gentlemen present, that we have the Continental Cholera amongst us? Those who are of this Opinion will hold up their Hands, when it was carried unanimously. Next, those who are of a contrary opinion, will hold up their hands, when not one Hand was held up.

A General Meeting of the *Board of Health*, was convened soon afterwards, and the following Resolution was drawn up by DR. BROWN, and agreed to unanimously.

" Resolved, that the Medical Gentlemen, under whose Observation Cases of C. Cholera have fallen, draw up a full Report of them, and place them, by the Forenoon of the 2nd. instant, in the Hands of Dr. Clanny, to be transmitted by him to the Board of Health of London."

This Report arrived in London on the 4th of November, when the Privy Council immediately ordered the Town of Sunderland to be placed in Quarantine.

As is the Duty of a Chairman I did not vote, nor could I, except a casting Vote had been needful.

These Facts remove from me the Odium, which some designing and ill-informed Men have propogated; and for these Facts, I have the original Documents in my possession. As the Organ of the Medical Department of the Board of Health of Sunderland, I have faithfully discharged my Duty between God and Man, and what I have performed has been barely Official, as Chairman of the Medical Department of the Board.

W. REID CLANNY, M. D.

Saturday Night, Nov. 12th, 1831.

H. J. Dixon, Printer, High Street, Bishopwearmouth.

teriologists, but in 1831 the government had to rely on sending down to Sunderland a physician who had seen the disease in Russia. His report settled the matter and everywhere new precautions were taken to keep the disease out. Other towns in County Durham announced that they would refuse to admit visitors from Sunderland, and many places, such as Edinburgh, posted guards on the roads to turn back 'trampers', who had walked from other towns and might be carrying the disease. Almost all the action taken, however, was carried out on local initiative, although the government did forbid shipping to sail from Sunderland to other ports, and sent down a 'half-pay' officer (an Army doctor living on half pay in between postings) who had fought a cholera epidemic in India, to help the local doctors.

The government was also still looking to the Almighty for help, and in March 1832 held a national day of fasting and humiliation, on which people were supposed to go to church to acknowledge their sins and to ask God in return to protect them from cholera. This proposal met with a good deal of mockery both in the House of Commons and outside; many people were beginning to suspect that it was human neglect that caused epidemics, rather than divine displeasure, and as one man later commented, 'the government was always getting the country into trouble and asking it to pray itself out of it'. Some communities, receiving so little help from the government, took the law into their own hands. At Cromarty, in the far north of Scotland, a town almost surrounded by water and so easy to protect, a public meeting decided to set up a local defence association, 'and ere midnight,' wrote its leader, 'our rounds and stations were marked out and our watches set'. The defence association posted sentries and organized a regular system of patrols to turn back 'all vagabonds and trampers'. Respectable travellers could hardly be shut out altogether so:

> it was ultimately agreed that . . . they should be first brought into a wooden building fitted up for the purpose and thoroughly fumigated with sulphur and chloride of lime . . . . A stranger well smoked came to be regarded as safe.

The great epidemic

Despite all the efforts to keep it out, cholera was soon appearing all over the North of England. By December it was in Newcastle where, according to the medical publication *The Lancet*, 'dropping cases now succeeded throughout the town'.

> The progress of the cholera is awful. It appears to be spreading in every direction . . . . The most terrific attack that I believe has occurred in Europe is at Gateshead. From one o'clock on Sunday (Christmas Day) to ten o'clock this day (45 hours) 119 persons have been seized and 52 have died.

Soon afterwards the disease appeared in nearby villages, in one of which, Newburn, 274 cases occurred — one person in every two in the population — and there were sixty-five deaths, or nearly one person in every eight.

Cholera first appeared in Scotland in mid-December. In January Edinburgh was infected and in February Glasgow, where there was the second most serious outbreak in the British Isles after London, with about 3,000 deaths. The disease eventually spread northwards, all through the Highlands, and even Cromarty, despite its 'smoking' of strangers, did not escape.

Meanwhile cholera had also been spreading southwards across England, and everywhere it was the dirtiest places which suffered most. Leeds, probably the filthiest city in the kingdom, lost 700 of its citizens, almost all of them in the unpaved and uncleansed parts of the town. Manchester, a larger place, suffered 900 deaths, fourteen of them in one wretched alley which became known as 'Cholera Court'. Liverpool, notorious

CHOLERA CONSULTATION
Long life to our Central Board — "in medio tutissimus ibis" — as we say in the Classics
I drink Reform in our Hospitals, may they close their doors against the public & the poor die in hackney coaches.
I pledge myself to keep some cases of Gout
May we preserve our health by bleeding the Country
Contagious Cholera
A Bad case
Cases made on the Shortest Notice
"Per varios casus, per tot discrimina rerum" Tendimus"
"By various cases & such discrimination we get on."
Dr. Bolus' Case Maker
New Case
New Case
Board & Lodging
Post Mortem Appearances — want of Employment Poverty Starvation Quarantine Stagnation Distress Blue Ruin —
While Drs differ & deny — The Country bleeds & patients die
Designed by A Bird
Drawn by G. Ck
Feby. 27th 1832 — Published by S Knights, Sweetings Alley Royal Exchange
THE CENTRAL BOARD of HEALTH

The dose to be repeated.
Emetic
Blue Pills
BOARD of HEALTH
STARVATION
Fee Fo Fum

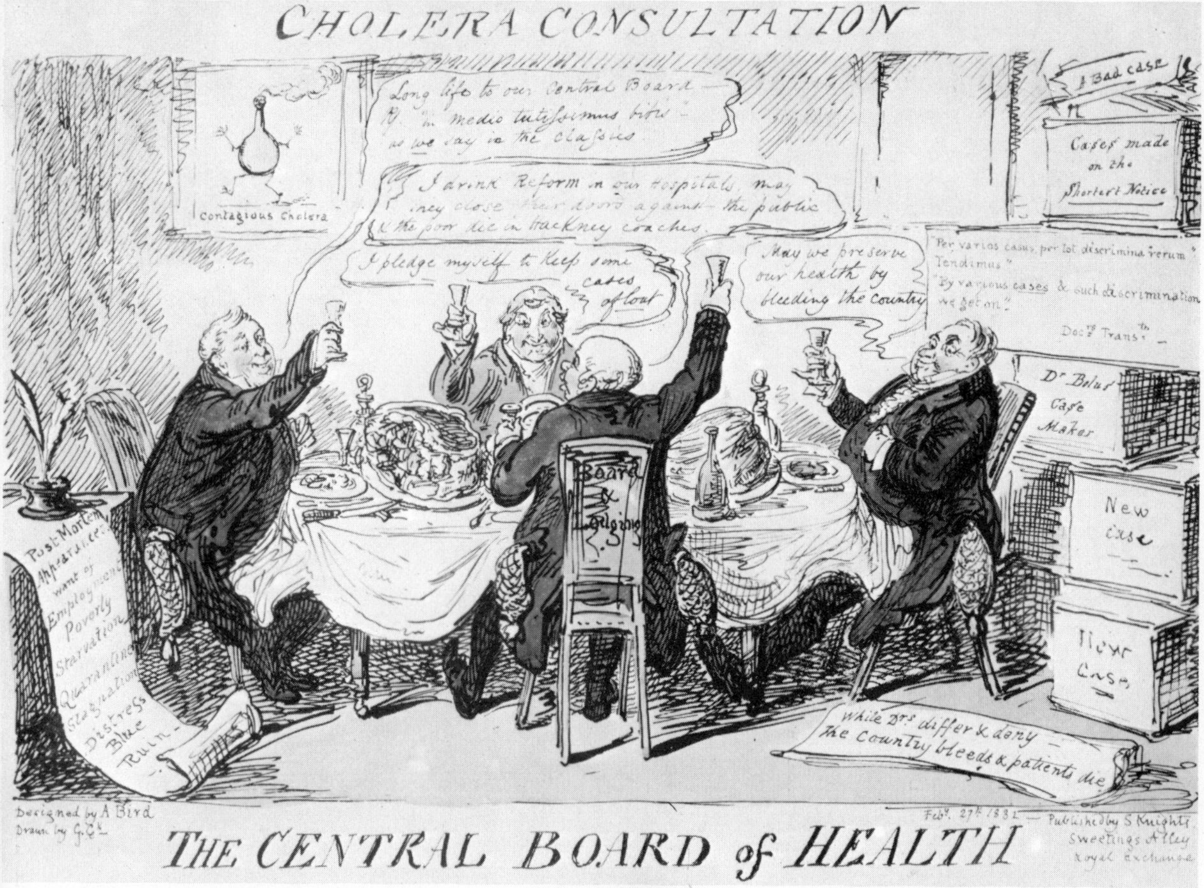

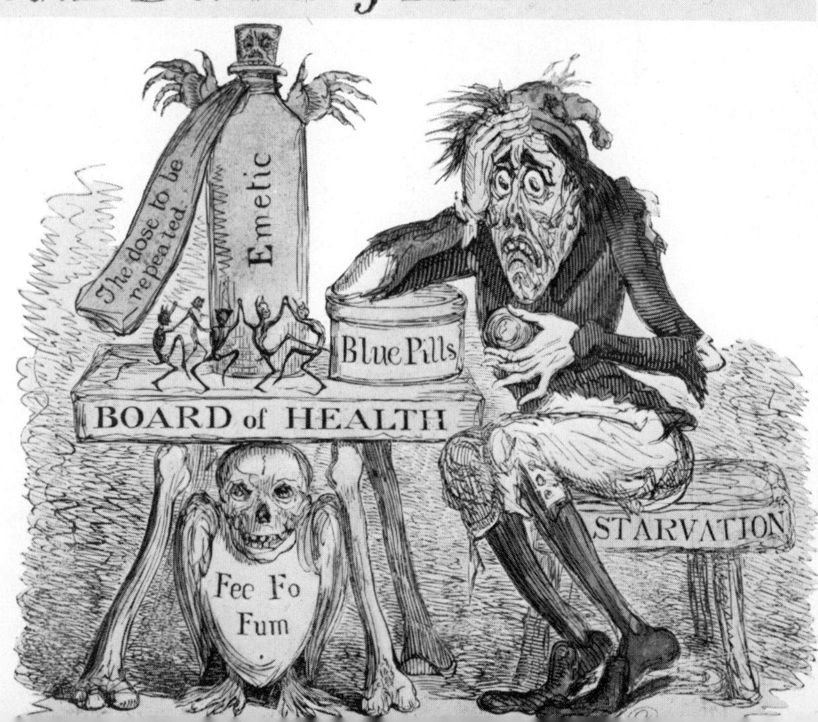

Two cynical views of the official arrangements to combat the cholera. In the first (above) cholera is represented on the wall as a smoking bomb, while fat doctors of the Central Board of Health toast one another with wine and gorge themselves on huge joints of meat. According to the second, if the cholera didn't get you, you were likely to lose out to the cures.

CHOLERA.

THE

DUDLEY BOARD OF HEALTH,

HEREBY GIVE NOTICE, THAT IN CONSEQUENCE OF THE

Church-yards at Dudley

Being so full, no one who has died of the CHOLERA will be permitted to be buried after *SUNDAY* next, (To-morrow) in either of the Burial Grounds of *St. Thomas's*, or *St. Edmund's*, in this Town.

All Persons who die from CHOLERA, must for the future be buried in the Church-yard at Netherton.

BOARD of HEALTH, DUDLEY.
September 1st, 1832.

W. MAURICE, PRINTER, HIGH STREET, DUDL

Cholera victims, according to the poster above, must be buried in Netherton; others could still be buried in Dudley. It is difficult to know whether the burial grounds really were full, or whether the Dudley Board of Health was anxious to get rid of cholera-infected bodies. Elsewhere the dread of cholera corpses was so great that there were rumours of people being buried before they had actually died.

In relation to its size Bilston was probably the worst hit town in England, with 745 dead, 131 widows and 450 orphans. A subscription raised the money for a special orphan school. The medal (below right) commemorates the opening, and the photograph (below left) shows the building as it really was.

One of the more extraordinary relics of the cholera epidemic of 1832 is the broadsheet, part of which is shown on the opposite page. It was sold for a penny, and the idea was apparently that friends and relatives of those who had died would pin it up on their walls as a memorial.

CHOLERA ORPHAN SCHOOL
OPENED AUGUST. 3. 1833
NUMBER OF ORPHANS
450
BY CHOLERA UNDER 12 YEARS OF AGE

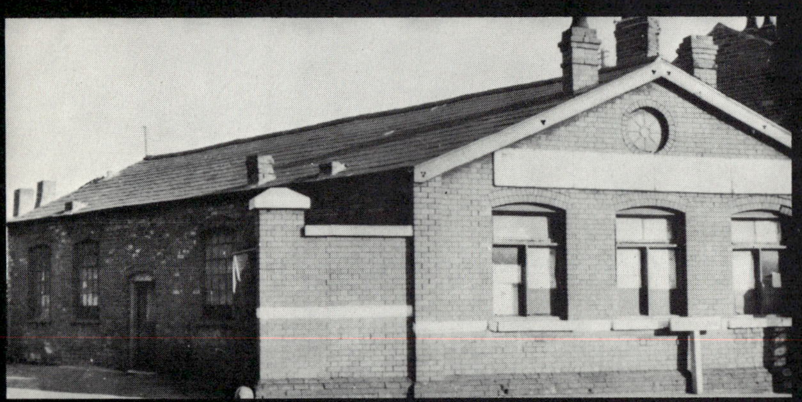

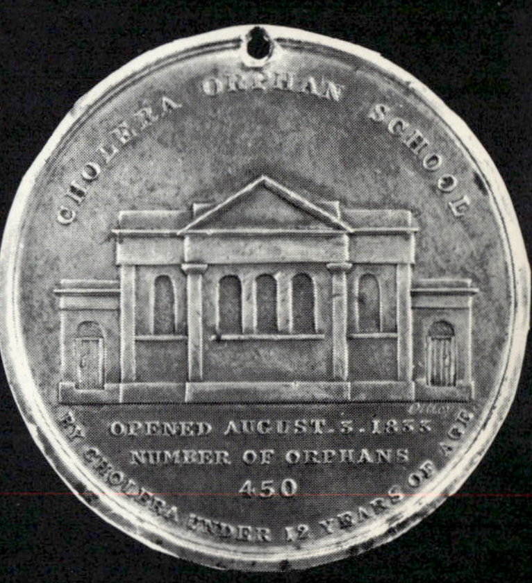

MEMORIAL

OF THE

CHOLERA,

WHICH VISITED BILSTON, IN THE YEAR OF OUR LORD, 1832.

TO meet the wishes of many of the friends and relatives of those who died by the awful visitation of CHOLERA, the following Statement (drawn up by a witness of these melancholy scenes,) is printed in a cheap form, to hang up in their houses as a MEMORIAL, for their children and future generations. When the Almighty is pleased to visit us with special judgments, or mercies, it is his most gracious design thereby, to correct our evils, to prevent our future misery, and to benefit and bless us. They who do not acknowledge his hand, who dislike to reflect on his dealings towards them, shew a bad state of mind. May the review of those scenes which some of us witnessed, and which are but faintly described in the following account, "So teach us to number our days, that we may apply our hearts unto wisdom."

THE CHOLERA

MADE its first appearance in England at Newcastle-upon-Tyne, and Sunderland, at the commencement of 1832; but it did not approach this Neighbourhood till the Month of June; and after raging at Tipton for several weeks, it then visited BILSTON, at the latter end of the Wake Week, and so rapid were its ravages, that before sufficient preparations could be made by the Board of Health, it assumed a very awful appearance. Elizabeth Dawson of Temple Street was [illegible] ho died, and [illegible] others in the same Street follow [illegible]

[illegible] nearly constant in attendance on funerals; as also was the Rev. J. Ham, at the Wesleyan burial ground: upwards of 400 were buried in the New Church Yard, and more than 300 in the Wesleyan Chapel Yard. Coffins could not be made fast enough in the Town, they were brought by cart-loads from Birmingham, and piled in heaps in the Hospital Yard, awaiting the last breath of their future tenants; about 40 were buried daily for some time; persons in health in the morning died at noon, and were buried at night. From August 3rd, to September 29th, there were no fewer th[illegible]

What call'd the young, the stout, the gay?
What was it snatch'd the old away?
What made such havoc in a day?
The Cholera.

What fill'd the people's minds with dread?
What made them sleepless on their bed?
What swell'd the numbers of the dead?
The Cholera.

What baffl'd all the Doctors' skill?
What did the Hospital so fill?
What was it made our Town so still?
The Cholera.

Cholera Statement.

Population of Bilston, in 1832	14,492
No. of Persons attacked by Cholera...	3,568
No. of Persons who died by Cholera,....	745
No. of Widowers who lost their Wives by Cholera,....................	103
No. of Widows who lost their Husbands by Cholera,....................	131
No. of Orphans under 12 years of age,..	450

The first Case August 3rd.
The last Case September 18th, 1832.
Amount of Subscriptions received,.. £ 8,536.

What led the people then to pray?
What did they meet for night and day?
What was the Lord to turn away?
The Cholera.

What, do we see a happier day?
What, have the people ceas'd to pray?
What now the Lord has turn'd away
The Cholera?

Come, let us all afresh repent,
Come, let us our whole hearts present,
Come, give them all to him who sent
The Cholera.

Reflections.

Ought we not to view the late fatal disease, which made such havoc amongst us, carrying away our friends and neighbours so rapidly, as a direct visitation of the Almighty? Should we not enquire whether the design of the Lord has been answered? Are we a more obedient and thankful people? Is there less Drunkenness, Sabbath-breaking, and such like disgraceful scenes of dissipation, and works of unrighteousness witnessed in our Streets? Shall we ever again hear of the cruel and inhuman practice of Bull-baiting? Were not amongst the first victims of Cholera, Drunkards, Bull-baiters, and characters of this description? We may forget the calls of the Almighty, we may harden our hearts, and impiously contemn the Lord; but 'woe unto him that striveth with his Maker!' We ought to feel grateful to God, who in the midst of death, preserved us alive; and we are this day 'the living, (may we be) the living to praise him.' During the Cholera, the House of God was considered a sanctuary,—his people the excellent of the earth,—and the means of grace esteemed and frequented. Why should it ever be otherwise? Oh! let each of us ever consider the salvation of our souls, 'the one thing needful.'

BILSTON:
Printed and Sold by Wm. Hackett, Market Place: Sold also by J. Etheridge, Church Street. Price One Penny

for its back-to-back and cellar dwellings, had 1,500 deaths, the largest number in England outside London. By August 1832, cholera was in the Midlands. The vicar of Bilston, near Wolverhampton, at the end of the month, wrote:

Since its appearance on the 3rd instant up to the present hour, 530 of the inhabitants have been swept away, which is as nearly as possible one twenty-seventh part of the population .... All kind of business is at a stand; nothing reigns here but want and disease, death and desolation.

In Exeter, in the far west, where 440 people died, the picture was almost as grim. A local doctor noted that:

In all quarters there were the sick, the dying and the dead. ... The general silence of the city, save when broken by the tolling of the funeral bell ... was most remarkable; the streets were deserted, the hurried steps of the medical men and their assistants, or of those running to seek their aid, alone were heard, while the one-horse hearse, occasionally passing on its duty, was almost the only carriage to be seen in the usually busy streets.

London suffered far more deaths than any other place in the British Isles — 5,300 officially, probably about 7,000 in fact, but here the disease caused less alarm. As one doctor wrote, rather cynically, in a medical magazine in September, it had inspired conversation rather than fear, since 'people talked about the cholera but they all knew ... its chief victims were "the poorest of the poor" ... and therefore there was never a real panic.' The 'poorest of the poor' had, of course, in those days when few working men had the vote, no one to speak up for them. Although one M.P. did draw attention to the case of a poor cholera patient who had been carried about London in a cab because no hospital would admit him, it was more the danger that middle-class people might become infected with the same disease through using the same vehicle that worried his fellow members than the sufferings of this unfortunate person. Some M.P.s complained about the overcrowded city graveyards, which had long been recognized as a public nuisance, and one protested that the inadequate ventilation in the House of Commons chamber might be endangering themselves, but on the whole neither back-benchers nor government were very worried about the voteless millions who needed protection.

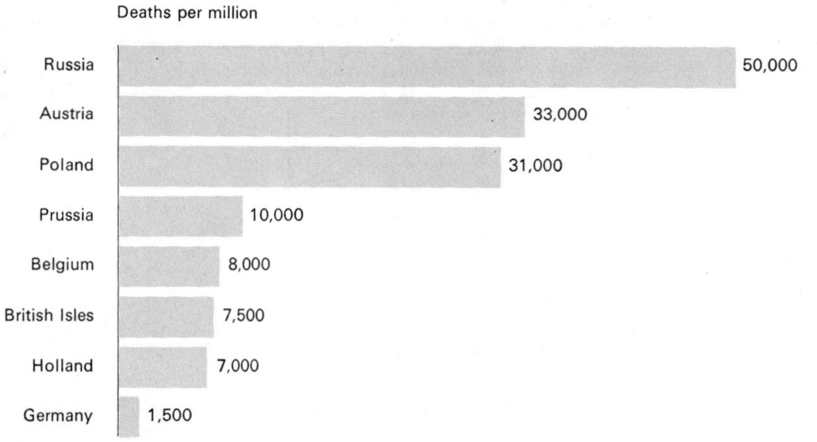

For all the panic caused by the epidemic, the British Isles were much better off than some other countries. This diagram shows how many people in every million died during the 1832 epidemic.

This cartoon shows doctors playing on the fear of cholera to obtain more fees.

Here is the real Cholera Morbus
that kil'ed all the people in India,
and was brought over by the survivers
PAY HERE
KILL OR CURE PHYSIC FOR THE CHOLERA ONLY 1 A DROP

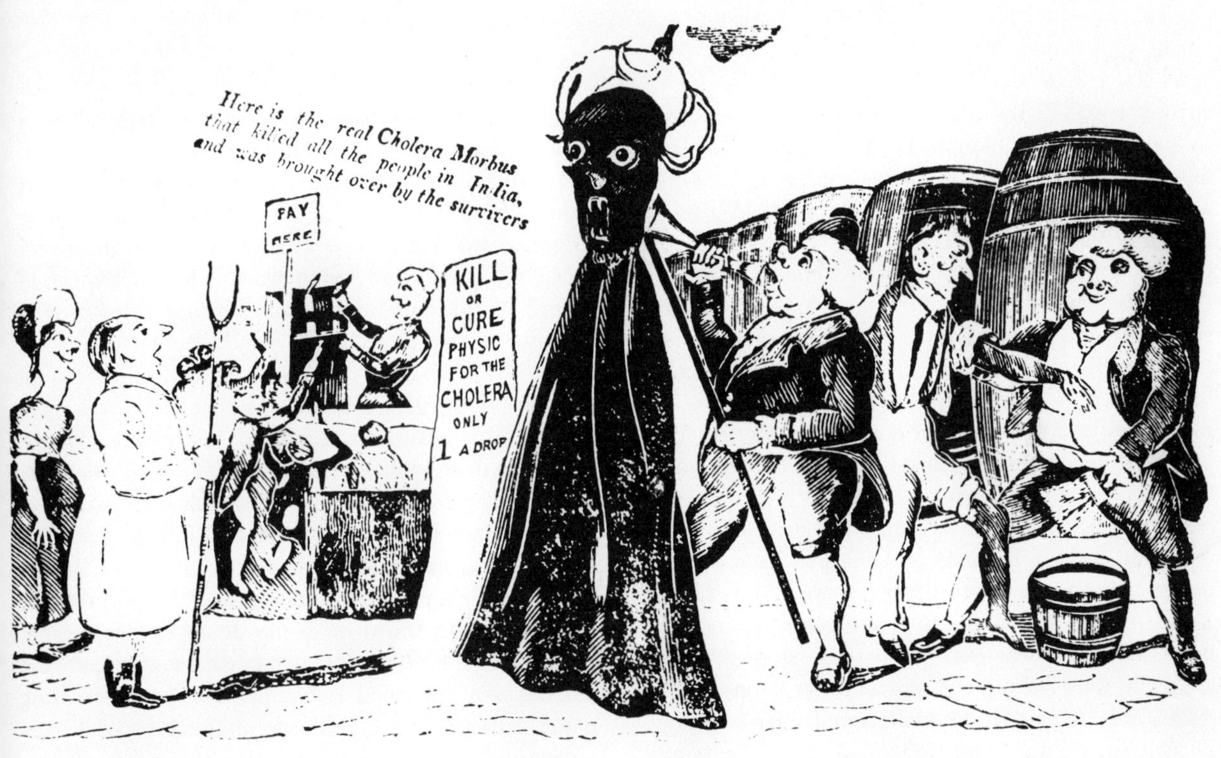

The doctors are powerless

Despite the attitude of the House of Commons, people who had actually seen the effects of cholera regarded it with terror, for not merely was it a new disease, which struck suddenly, and which the doctors obviously had no idea how to cure, but it spread mysteriously in a way no one could understand. As a result, many people, like the businessmen of Sunderland, preferred to pretend that it did not exist at all. A ballad was actually told on the streets of London alleging that news of the disease was a hoax 'to raise the doctors' stuff', i.e. to make money for the medical profession, and a cartoon appeared in a weekly paper showing a doctor painting a healthy man black to make him look as though he had cholera. But no one who had actually seen the disease was under any illusion about it. A doctor who had treated many cases in Sunderland described how the first sign that one had caught cholera might be:

> giddiness, ringing in the ears, uneasiness . . . followed by a prickly sensation in the arms and legs, extending sometimes to the fingers and toes; the hands and feet become cold and bedewed with a copious clammy moisture. . . . The moment the patient moves . . . he is either sick or purged.

This first purging probably involved 'a prodigious evacuation, when the whole intestines seem to be emptied at once', and it was followed by violent diarrhoea and vomiting in which the body lost several pints of fluid in a few minutes, expelled as if from a syringe. The doctor might find the bedclothes saturated and the floor of the bedroom awash. The loss of fluid from the body caused the skin and finger nails to turn blue or black and caused the patient to look shrunken and shrivelled, until he resembled, according to one doctor, a monkey rather than a man. Later he felt the pain of 'cramps' in his fingers or toes and across his chest, as if he was 'being screwed through with a screw' until, worn out but still conscious, the patient would collapse, fall into a coma and die.

In the crowded hovels of the poor, lacking privacy, sanitation and a water supply, few diseases could have been more horrible, but most people were unwilling to be removed to hospital and would only go as a last resort, so that the hospital doctors usually received only the most hopeless cases. In Manchester, where the people had 'an unconquerable horror' of cholera hospitals, nearly half those admitted died and in the excellent cholera hospital in Glasgow, in a disused police station, the mortality rate was 70 per cent. Such figures increased the prejudice against the hospitals and desperately ill people being removed to them were sometimes 'rescued' by angry mobs. At St Marylebone, in London, a mob carried off one patient in triumph, and threatened the bearers and surgeons, and in Manchester, *The Times* reported, 'a mob numbering several thousand persons . . . broke into the hospital, carried off the patients to their homes and wrecked the furniture and fittings of the wards. The military was at length called out to clear the streets.' (One Irish nurse who could not escape in time 'jumped into a bed . . . covered herself up and began to writhe and groan, as if suffering from cholera', thus escaping attack.)

Similar disorders, though for different reasons, occurred in other parts of the British Isles. One woman suffering from cholera who struggled five miles to a village in Clackmannanshire in Scotland to take refuge with her mother was dragged from her bed by the angry villagers and sent back in a cart to die, and next morning the terrified villagers burned the mother's cottage to the ground. Two doctors who diagnosed the first case of cholera in Ireland, in a suburb of Dublin, 'escaped injury almost by a miracle. . . . A furious mob of men, women and children hurled stones, mud, brickbats at them from all sides. Their carriage was battered and broken by the missiles.' It was widely believed that the doctors were deliberately killing any patients unwise enough to go into hospital in order to use their bodies for dissection – corpses for research were at this time almost unobtainable through normal means and, very sensibly, many doctors did perform post-mortems to try and discover more about the disease. In Exeter the mayor actually found it necessary to issue a handbill warning the public against 'the unfounded and uncharitable prejudice which has been evinced towards the medical practitioners', threatening 'heavy fines and imprisonment' for anyone who interfered with the work of the Board of Health, but even so the *Western Times* reported that one doctor had become 'alarmed for his personal safety' after being called in the street 'one of the gang of bloody murderers who did all the mischief'.

The doctors did not deserve their unpopularity. Most of them had worked tirelessly and heroically to help their patients, for precious little reward in return. Five medical students who had daily risked their lives fighting the Bilston epidemic received only five guineas each; a public subscription for the doctors in Exeter raised less than £250. No wonder one doctor caustically observed that 'thanks are indeed forthcoming, for they cost nothing'. But it was true that the doctors were little wiser about cholera at the end of the epidemic than at the beginning. No one knew what caused it; no one knew how it spread and only the most foolish and conceited even claimed to be able to cure it. The *Glasgow Medical Journal* spoke for the whole profession when it declared in May 1832 that the recommended drugs would 'be found, one and all, equally impotent to arrest the course of that merciless distem-

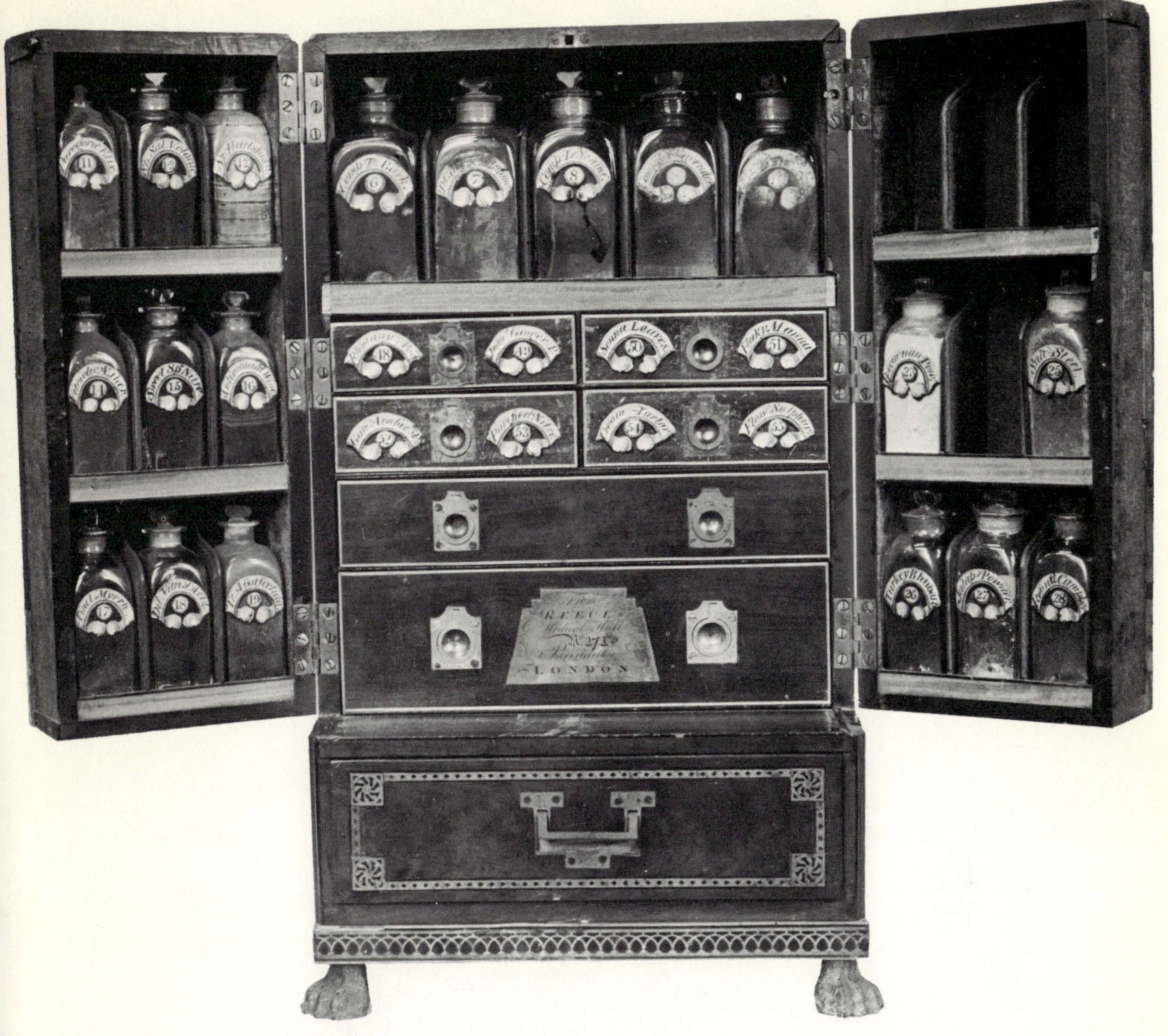

A nineteenth-century domestic medicine chest.

per. We have to tell our readers . . . that perhaps they had better stand quietly by . . . and give nature and the disease a fair field for the combat.'

But most doctors were not willing to lose a patient without a struggle and every type of treatment was tried. Some doctors favoured cold water and ice to drag the system back from collapse; others preferred hot compresses and baths. One who introduced hot air into his patient's bed to warm him was so successful that he set it on fire, while another tried an even more novel method, electricity, but all his patients died, either, according to him, because the battery ran out or because they shook off the contact wires. One of the commonest treatments was bleeding which, as in

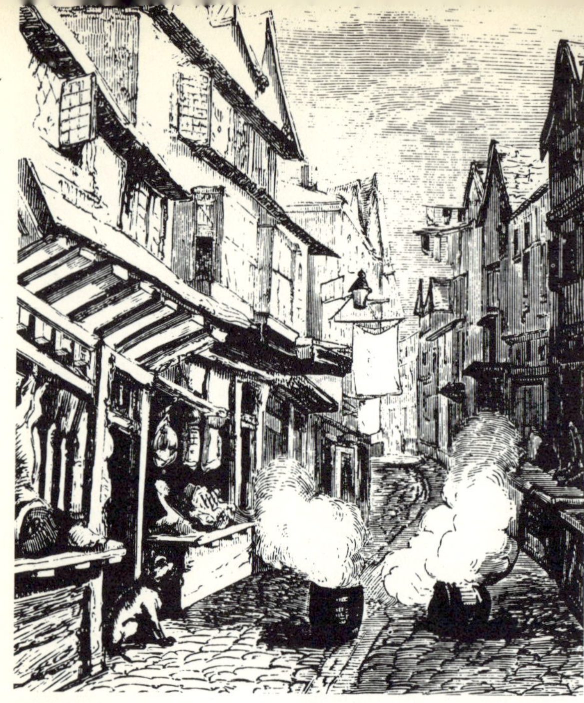

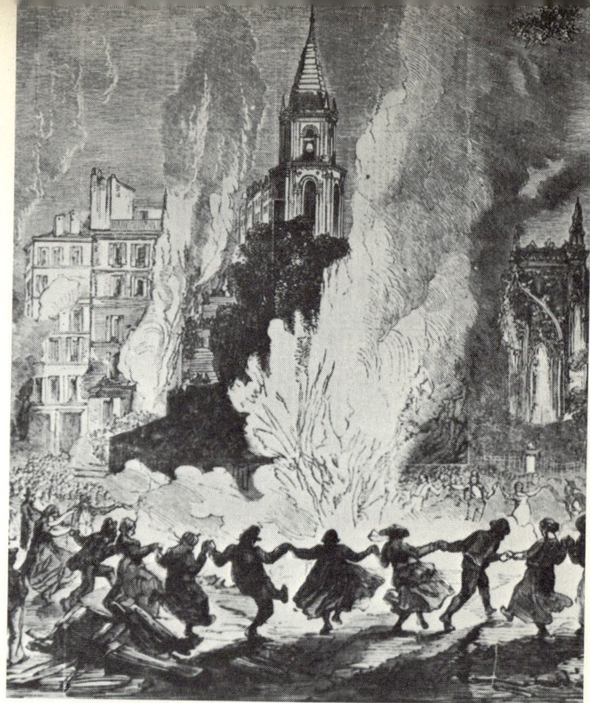

A favourite theory was that the pestilence could be smoked out. The picture on the left above shows tar barrels being burnt in Exeter; on the right, bonfires in Marseilles. Below is a French engraving of passengers being fumigated with strong carbolic acid. An important part of people's thinking about medical matters was that if something was unpleasant for human beings, it was pretty well bound to be unpleasant for the disease. The more unpleasant, the more effective the treatment was likely to be. Actually, this was quite untrue, but it probably did something to help people's peace of mind.

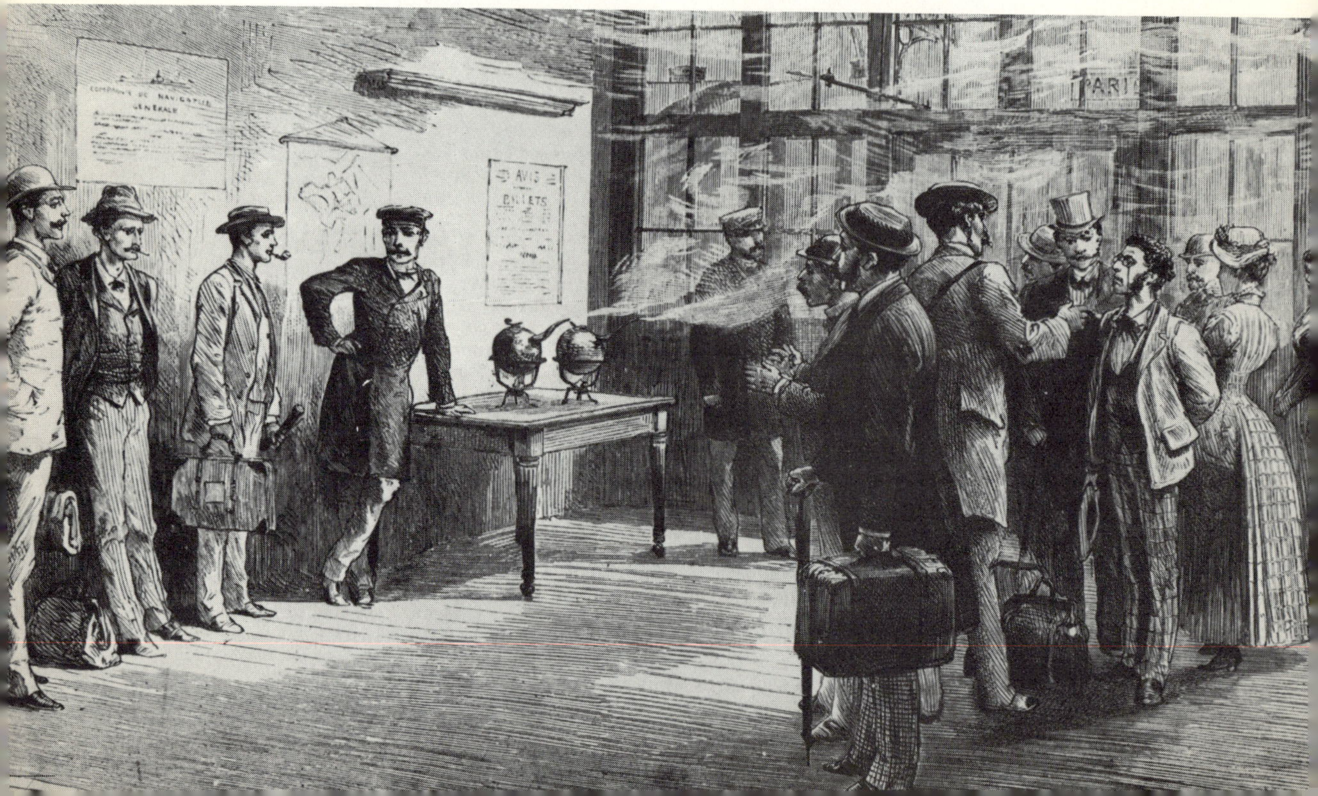

other illnesses, was believed to relieve the pressure on the patient's system while draining off some of his supposedly infected blood. One leaflet advised having thirty leeches in the house to suck your blood, just in case you caught cholera, and most doctors had their lancet out ready to open a vein and draw off up to twenty-four fluid ounces of blood almost before their bags were unpacked. A Penzance doctor recommended an incision in the patient's head 'to relieve oppression of the brain', but the two unfortunate people on whom he tried his method died.

Doctors at that time had, of course, far fewer drugs to choose from and in dealing with cholera relied mainly on two old favourites, opium and calomel, a compound of mercury. Since there was no systematic research and clinical trial of new drugs, of which in any case none had been produced for years, many doctors were prepared to try almost any substance once. Some experimented with small doses of arsenic 'to clear out the patient's body of infection' by giving him even more violent diarrhoea, others, on the same theory, prescribed mustard and water to make him even more sick. Other 'drugs' which were tried included tobacco, burnt cork, horse radish, black pepper and pounded ginger. They had, however, one thing in common; none of them worked.

On the wings of the air

No one knew how cholera spread. In some European countries there had been peasant risings against the nobility who were suspected of poisoning the wells and rivers to keep the population down. In England the medical profession itself was divided into two main groups, the contagionists and the miasmatists. The contagionists believed that, like measles, cholera spread by physical contact with a sick person, or his clothes or bedding, which explained why outbreaks were so often concentrated in one district or street. The miasmatists, on the other hand, thought that cholera was due to an infection lurking in dirt or stagnant water, which was touched off by some special atmospheric conditions of temperature, or humidity, or some unidentified agent like 'the electric fluid'. This theory explained both the disease's preference for ill-ventilated and ill-cleaned places and its mysterious appearance in scattered places many miles apart. During the next few years tremendous efforts were made to substantiate these theories. The miasmatists took innumerable readings of temperature and atmospheric pressure to try to find the precise combination of conditions which released the fatal 'miasma' on the air. One flew a kite with a loaf and some meat and fish attached to it in a cholera-affected area and said that as they were bad when he hauled them down this 'proved' that infected air was to blame. The contagionists spent thousands of hours tracing the course of every isolated outbreak to try to establish some contact with a previous epidemic. With the general public, the theory that cholera travelled, as one doctor put it, 'on the wings of the air' gained wide acceptance. In towns attacked by cholera tar barrels or heaps of tobacco were often burned to kill the supposed infection and sometimes people danced round huge bonfires as if celebrating a holiday. The *Lancet* referred scornfully to one Persian town where the inhabitants tried to frighten the cholera away with 'a singular sanitory measure.... Salvoes of artillery and peals of musketry roared from the rising to the setting sun, loud shouts were raised by united thousands and gongs and trumpets increased the horrid commotion.' Englishmen had, however, little cause to feel superior. A London dentist wrote an open letter to the government urging them to set up cannon around London and to fire them off every hour for the purpose of 'disinfecting the atmosphere'.

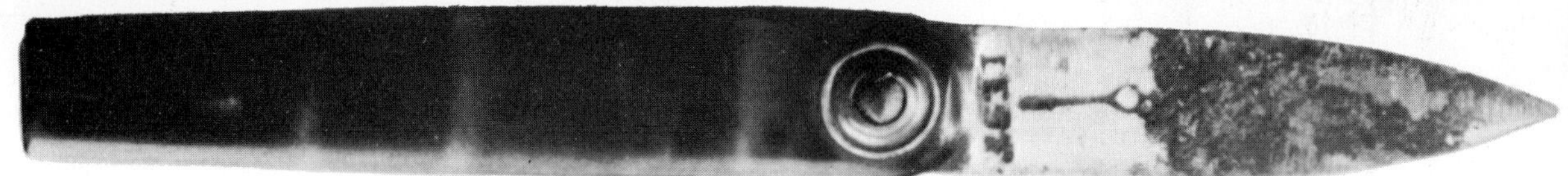

The traditional method of treatment for almost anything was bleeding. Usually a scalpel would be used for this, but leeches were enjoying a revival at this time in England

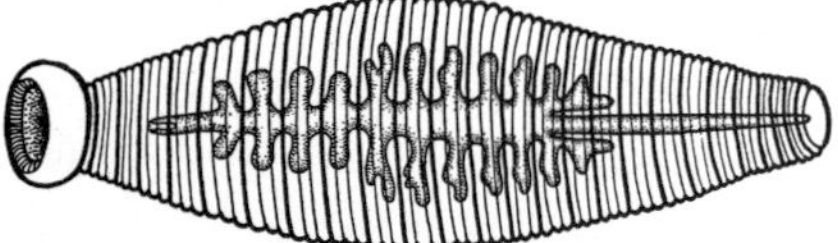

and on the continent: forty-one million leeches were imported into France in 1833. They had been popular with the medical profession during the seventeenth century, but their use had declined in the eighteenth. (Wordsworth, the poet, recalls meeting a leech gatherer in the Lake District in 'Resolution and Independence'.) The leeches were usually applied, up to ten at a time, on the back of the patient. To ensure that the leech extracted as much blood as possible, the tail would sometimes be cut off. In this way the leech would pump the patient's blood through himself before dying of exhaustion.

Other popular techniques were purging with laxatives or with drugs to make the patient vomit. At the same time the patient would often be put on a diet, possibly a starvation diet. It was a hard business being ill in the early nineteenth century. Knowledge about many illnesses was so sketchy that most doctors had their own pet theories about the way to threat them. The best you could hope for was that your doctor believed more in drugs such as opium or calomel than in bleeding, vomiting or starving.

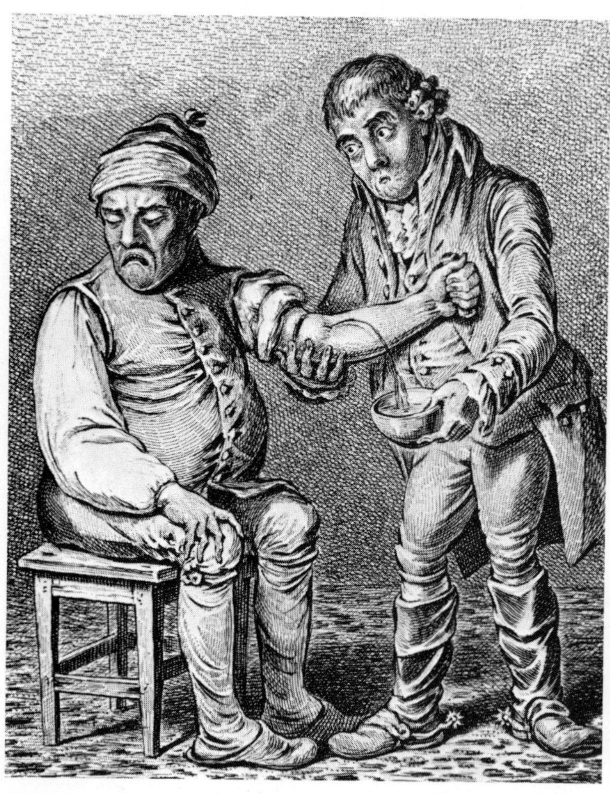

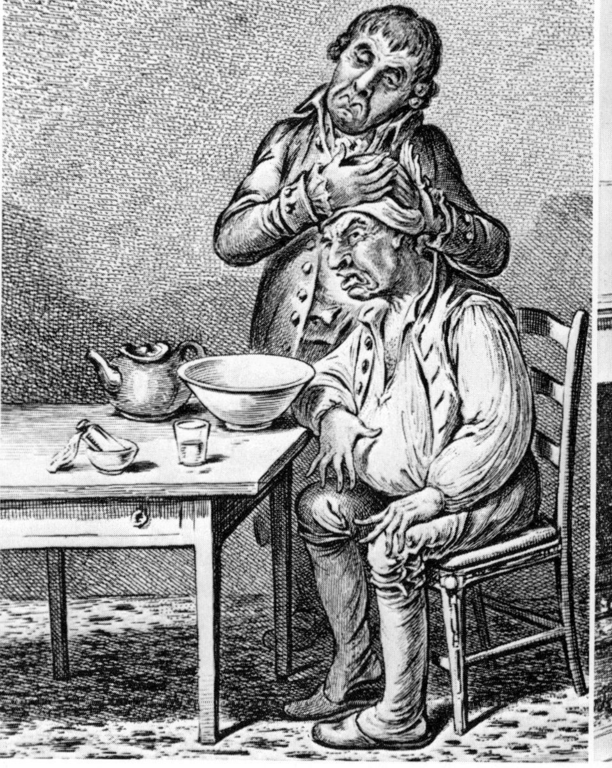

A public-spirited surgeon issued this poster on the treatment of cholera during the 1832 epidemic. Public-spirited he may have been, but his method of treatment would have been virtually useless.

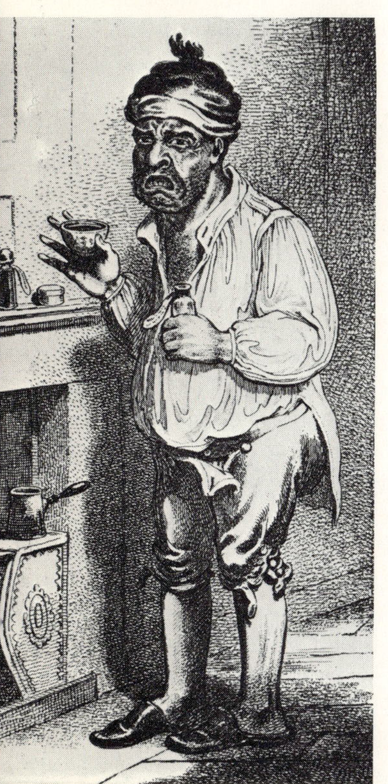

A cynical view of the fate of the patient, by James Gillray: bleeding, purging and (on the right) taking some very nasty medicine.

Free Hospital for the Cure of Malignant Diseases,

Greville Street, Hatton Garden.

MALIGNANT CHOLERA.

THERE are two stages in this Disease ; the Symptoms of both are as follows :—

The First Stage.—A feeling of general weakness over the whole body, sickness with pain about the stomach, purging and twitching pains in the bowels, a clammy feeling in the mouth, and a desire to drink more than usually. These symptoms constitute the first stage of the disorder ; and in some persons they will continue for several days, but in others they quickly run into the Second Stage.

Second Stage.—This is known by the weakness becoming extreme,—vomiting and purging of watery fluid greatly increased,—extreme thirst,—cramps in the hands, feet, and legs,—coldness of all the limbs,—cold breath, —sunken eyes,—dark blue appearance of the extremities,—and no pulsation is perceptible at the wrist. In Children the signs are vomiting, purging, great thirst, and general restlessness.

The disease during the first stage may always be cured ; but if neglected and allowed to pass into the second stage, it is fatal in three out of four cases. At this Hospital not one patient has been lost when admitted during the first stage of the complaint ; and many have been saved by great attention to medicine even in the second stage. The treatment is very simple, and the medicines can be procured at a very cheap rate.

Remedies during the First Stage.—For Children up to four years old :

Calomel, five grains.
Ginger, five grains.

Mixed together for a dose. This powder to be given immediately, mixed in a little treacle : and two hours after the powder, give the following draught :

Powdered Rhubarb, ten grains.
Castor Oil, half an ounce.

Mixed together, and given in half a small cup of strong coffee.
Should the vomiting and purging continue, give two table spoonsful of soda water every half hour, and repeat the powder of calomel and ginger four hours after the draught.

From the age of four years to fourteen, give the following powder and draught after the same manner :

Calomel, nine grains.
Ginger, nine grains —Mix'd.

The draught:

Castor Oil, three quarters of an ounce.
Tincture of Rhubarb, two drachms.
Powdered Rhubarb, eight grains.—Mix'd.

From the age of fourteen and upwards, take the following powder and draught :

Calomel, fifteen grains, to twenty.
Ginger, fifteen grains, to twenty.—Mix'd.

The draught :—

Castor Oil, and
Tincture of Rhubarb, of each one ounce.—Mix'd.

Small draughts of soda water to be taken by all, providing the vomiting continues ; and, should the symptoms not abate, the powder and draught may be repeated four hours after the first dose. Strong beef tea, well seasoned with salt and pepper, may be taken during the progress of the disease ; but the patient must strictly avoid drinking a quantity of any fluid whatsoever at this period. Providing these remedies fail in removing the disorder, and the Second-Stage ensues, the following plan must be rigidly observed, it being the only one yet known that has restored a single patient ; it is on the principle of the saline treatment suggested by Dr. Stephens :—

For Children up to the age of four years, . { Common Salt, one scruple. / Carbonate of Soda, six grains. / Oxymuriate of Potash, two grains.—Mix, for one dose.

From four to fourteen years of age, . . { Common Salt, one drachm. / Carbonate of Soda, ten grains. / Oxymuriate of Potash, three grains.—Mix.

For persons above the age of fourteen years, { Common Salt, two drachms. / Carbonate of Soda, one scruple. / Oxymuriate of Potash, seven grains.—Mix.

The above powders to be given every quarter of an hour, dissolved in a small quantity of cold water. During this treatment, as much cold water or weak beef tea may be taken as the patients desire ; the more the better.

The above are the only remedies now used during the progress of the disorder in this Hospital, with the addition of hot salt-water bathing ; and such has been the success, that I feel it my duty to advise the same to the inhabitants of the adjoining parishes, but more particularly to that of St. Martin's, Ludgate, it being that portion of the City Liberty, in Farringdon Without, which is appropriated to my charge by the City Board of Health ; and any person desiring further information may receive it gratuitously any day at One o'clock, at this Hospital ; or before Ten o'clock in the Morning, at my residence, No. 2, Thavies Inn, Holborn-hill.

WILLIAM MARSDEN, Surgeon.

Greville Street Free Hospital for the Cure of Malignant Diseases,
July 20th, 1832.

N.B. Persons not able to pay for medicines will be furnished with them free, by applying as above directed. Should any case occur, it is requested that notice be immediately sent to the Surgeon, who will superintend the above plan of treatment.

Printed by Richard Taylor, Red Lion Court, Fleet Street.

3 The great diseases and the sanitary movement

The diseases that killed

Cholera was a frightening disease. It struck fast, usually fatally, and nobody could tell where (or perhaps more important *who*) it would strike next. But cholera was an epidemic disease — that is to say, it broke out unpredictably, spread, and eventually died down. It might break out again, but the number dying from the disease was never constant from year to year.

What were the diseases that yearly took their toll of the population? The first Act for the registration of births, marriages and deaths in England and Wales did not come into effect until 1837. Before that, according to an article in the *Lancet* of 1848, 'a perfect chaos respecting population mortality reigned'. For this reason it is difficult to obtain figures for the main diseases and causes of death in the early part of the nineteenth century. By the middle of the century, however, more and more districts were keeping detailed records of mortality and its causes. In 1858, Edward Greenhow, a lecturer on public health at St Thomas's Hospital, compared these figures over the whole country. His report is a good guide to the state of the nation's health during the 1840s and 1850s. Greenhow showed that a great deal of disease over the years 1848–55 had been directly caused by bad sanitary conditions. The average annual death rate per 100,000 of the population was 2,266 and of these only a tenth were due simply to old age. Children, being particularly vulnerable, were 'a sensitive test of sanitary circumstances'. Three quarters of the deaths from infectious diseases were children under five years of age.

The white plague

The most consistent and dangerous disease was tuberculosis or T.B., then called consumption. Sometimes known as 'the white plague', or more poetically, as the 'captain of the armies of death', tuberculosis accounted for more deaths than any other disease. T.B. eats away the lungs so that a patient becomes frail and wastes away, coughs a great deal and spits blood frequently. When this happened people spoke of a friend 'going into a decline', but sometimes the disease carried the victim off by a sudden attack, resembling pneumonia, and was called 'galloping consumption'. T.B. so often attacked people in the same family that some doctors believed it was inherited, and as so many writers, painters and musicians suffered from it some doctors wondered if artistic people were particularly susceptible to the disease. In fact it attacked all classes, though the worst sufferers were people in the poorest quarters of the great cities, living in airless, overcrowded slums, with no money to spare for special medicines, good food and rest in a healthy climate.

Typhoid fever

Apart from cholera, the other great 'dirt disease' of nineteenth-century England was typhoid, or enteric fever, which also spreads through contaminated water and food and which particularly attacks young people in their teens. The disease began with nose-bleeding and a high temperature, went on to pink spots on the skin, diarrhoea and delirium, and often ended in death through complications like intestinal bleeding. While cholera attacked in sudden epidemics, typhoid killed five or ten thousand victims year after year and it was far slower to leave the British Isles. The 'apostle of sanitation', John Simon, described a sudden outbreak of typhoid in Essex in 1867, where

> in a village of only nine hundred inhabitants and for the most part within a period of two months, fully three hundred persons were attacked with typhoid fever, and forty-one of the number died. . . . This most calamitous visitation, was [said Simon] due solely to conditions of local filth.

As late as the 1890s typhoid was still killing 6,000 people a year in the British Isles.

Suppose the idea of vaccination was a totally new one to you. Suppose then that some doctors began to say that people could be protected from a serious disease by being given it. Would *you* allow your child to be vaccinated? True, these doctors were only suggesting that your child be given cowpox, which was much less serious than smallpox itself, but the idea still seemed a very strange and frightening one. This cartoon – one of many – gives some idea about how strongly people felt about vaccination in the early nineteenth century.

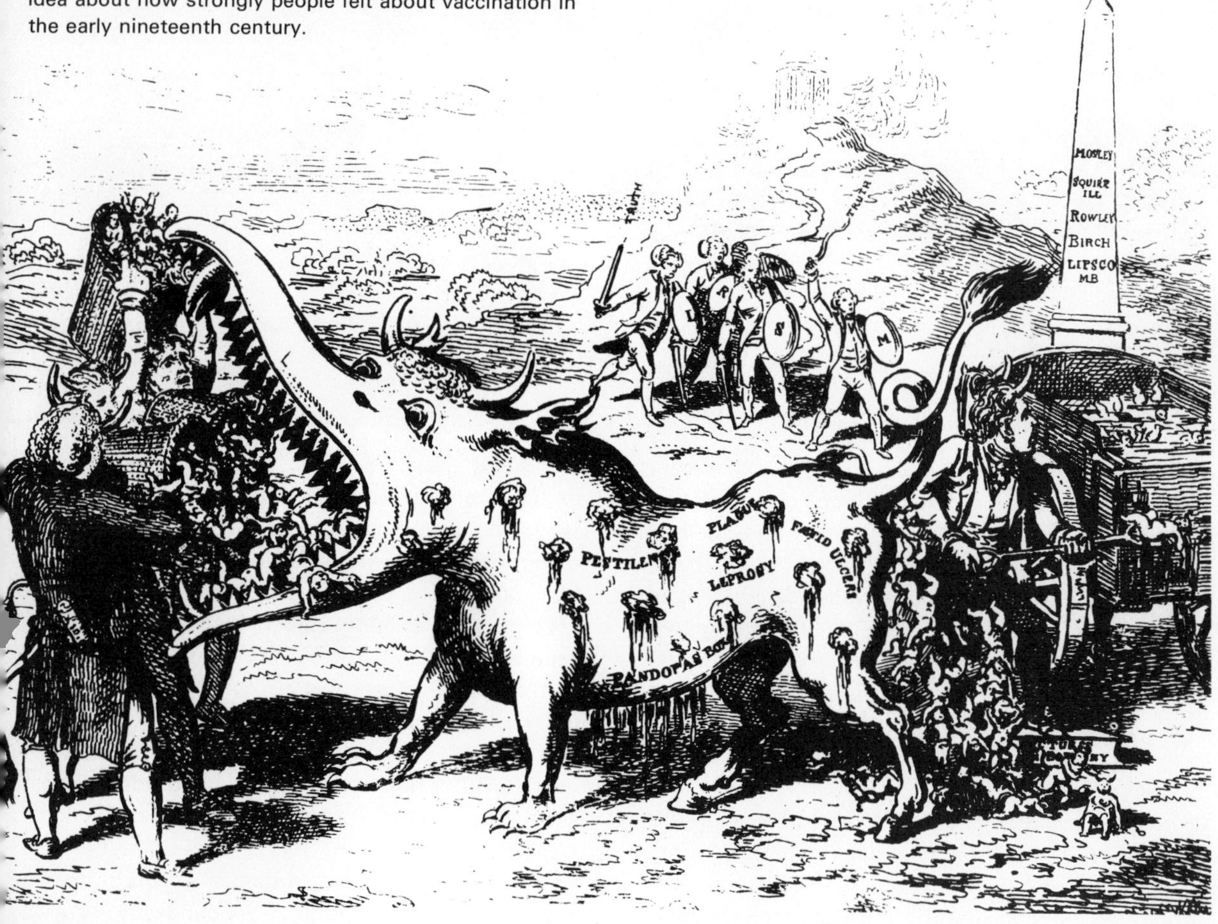

Smallpox

Smallpox was also a disease which killed large numbers of people every year. But in this case the continuing dangerousness of the disease was surprising. At the end of the eighteenth century, a country doctor by the name of Edward Jenner had heard that there was a belief among country people that you would not contract smallpox if you had had cowpox, a similar but much less serious disease. Jenner found that by deliberately giving a small boy cowpox he could immunize him against smallpox. This method of treatment, which came to be known as vaccination, we shall return to later. But sixty years after Jenner's discovery of vaccination, deaths from smallpox could still amount to one quarter of the deaths in certain districts. The vast majority of victims had either not been properly vaccinated, or not vaccinated at all. As the Medical Officer to the Board of Health re-

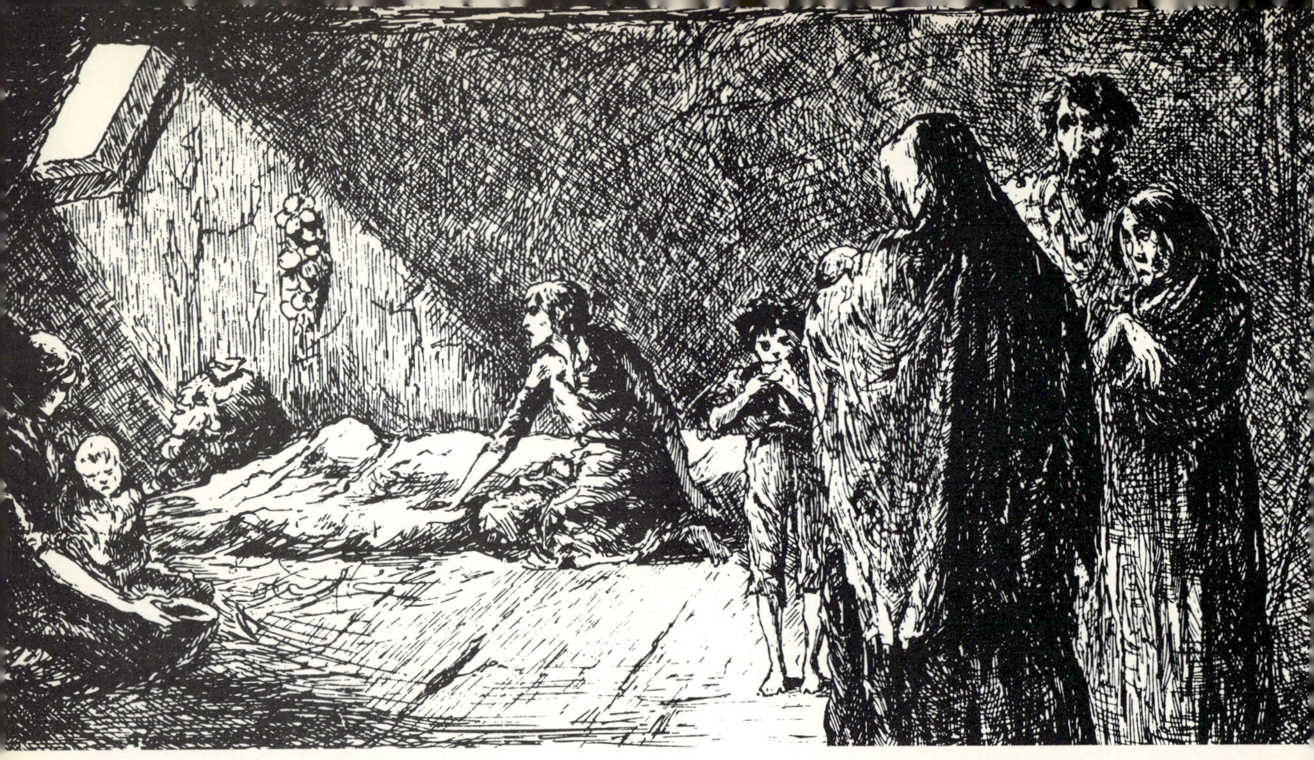

marked, 'To foreign nations, who have learnt from us the means of preventing smallpox, it must seem almost incredible that we still annually suffer four or five thousand deaths by the disease.'

A smaller number of deaths were caused by ague (malarial fever), nervous convulsions or 'fits', scurvy and 'insanity' — which included paralysis and epilepsy. Here too, overcrowding, bad diet and exhaustion helped to weaken and depress the patient.

Children and disease

All in all, the major diseases of the early nineteenth century have two things in common: they are either diseases caused or encouraged by unsanitary conditions and poor food and air, or they are diseases that particularly affect children and young people, or both. The infantile mortality rate — the number of deaths of infants under the age of one year for every thousand births — is a good index of the health of a town or country, and anyone who looks at the gravestones in an old churchyard will soon see for himself what a high proportion of deaths occurred in childhood. In Liverpool in 1840 the infantile death rate was 23 per cent; even in rural Wiltshire it was 16 per cent. In his great *Report* in 1842 Edwin Chadwick noted that 'It is an appalling fact that, of all who are born of the labouring classes in Manchester, more than 57 per cent die before they attain five years of age' — adding characteristically, 'that is, before they can be engaged in factory labour.' As late as 1901, in England and Wales, the infantile mortality rate was still 151; by 1916 it was down to 91, by 1945 to 46 and by 1965 — the sharpest drop of all — to 19. The death rate today from the common infectious diseases of childhood is now only one two-hundredth part of what it was in 1850.

Apart from diseases like typhoid, which also attacked adults, the greatest danger to children came for many years from diphtheria which, beginning with a sore throat, often led to blood poisoning and heart failure, and to the growth of a membrane or skin across the tonsils which might choke the patient to death. Doctors treating diphtheria patients often had to perform the operation of tracheotomy, or cutting of the throat, to enable the patient to breathe, and when there was no time to call the doctor, nurses sometimes did this themselves with a pen-knife or even a hat-pin.

A dead body left under a sheet in the family living-room before burial.

Cleaning up after cholera

Clean up the water supply, reform the street drainage and house sewerage systems, improve their diet, re-house the poorer members of the population — do all this and consumption, typhoid, and cholera might not disappear, but they would certainly be much reduced. Many doctors understood this, even though they could not tell exactly how a disease like cholera spread. Much sensible work had been done in the late eighteenth and early nineteenth century, but this was mainly directed towards the improvement of conditions in the army and navy. (Ironically, authorities were quick to do something about sanitary conditions when it meant that the efficiency of fighting forces might be affected.) But almost nothing was done about towns, and the towns were getting worse every year as the population swelled. This is where cholera came in. It was cholera that counted. You could become used to tens of thousands of people dying each year of consumption or typhoid, but something as dramatic and terrifying and sudden as the Asiatic cholera was a different matter entirely.

Whatever their ideas about the way cholera spread, doctors all agreed that it was concentrated in the most unsanitary places. When the first epidemic finally died out in 1833, after killing about 60,000 people, there was a drive in many places to clean up the streets and alleys. Enthusiasm was naturally greatest in places which had suffered most from cholera. In Exeter there was a public competition for schemes to provide a new water supply and before long thirteen miles of new sewers had also been laid, while the Leeds Board of Health sent a report on the insanitary state of their city to the Home Secretary with a resolution that:

> As the facts . . . are applicable to all large towns . . . this Board is of opinion that a general Act of Parliament for sewering, draining, cleaning and paving would prove a public benefit.

But the government was not yet ready to take such a drastic step and during the next few years the pressure for improvement came largely from public-spirited private individuals and progressive Members of Parliament. The key figure in what became known as 'the sanitary movement' was a civil servant, Edwin Chadwick, who has already been mentioned. Chadwick was a dry, humourless, unsociable man; he could not get on with children and he usually ended up by quarrelling with his adult colleagues, but he was a man of great energy, enterprise and vision. After training as a barrister and working as a journalist, he was thirty-two when he became a civil servant in 1832. When the government in 1834 set up its Poor Law Board, to run the new system of workhouses, Chadwick became its secretary. He first became interested in public health because of the cost of supporting the thousands of widows and orphans who were left destitute every year when men died in the prime of life from diseases which he believed to be preventable. In 1838 he carried out a great survey of the poor districts of East London where cholera had struck hardest six years before, and soon afterwards Parliament set up the first Select Committee on the Health of Towns.

In 1842 Chadwick's greatest work was published, *The Report on the Sanitary Condition of the Labouring Population*. This is the most important document in the history of public health. Its 457 pages were crammed with 'sanitary maps' showing how diseases like cholera were concentrated in the worst drained parts of cities, tables of statistics explaining how the expectation of life varied in different places, and practical suggestions for improving matters. Chadwick believed that there should be a unified system of sanitary control, with one body responsible for *all* sanitary matters in any town, and he worked out that every family could be given a decent house,

A group of industrial cottages in Preston in 1844. The privies are at the end of the yards and drain into an open trench which runs down the middle. The landlord cleaned the trench out twice a year and piled the contents near by.

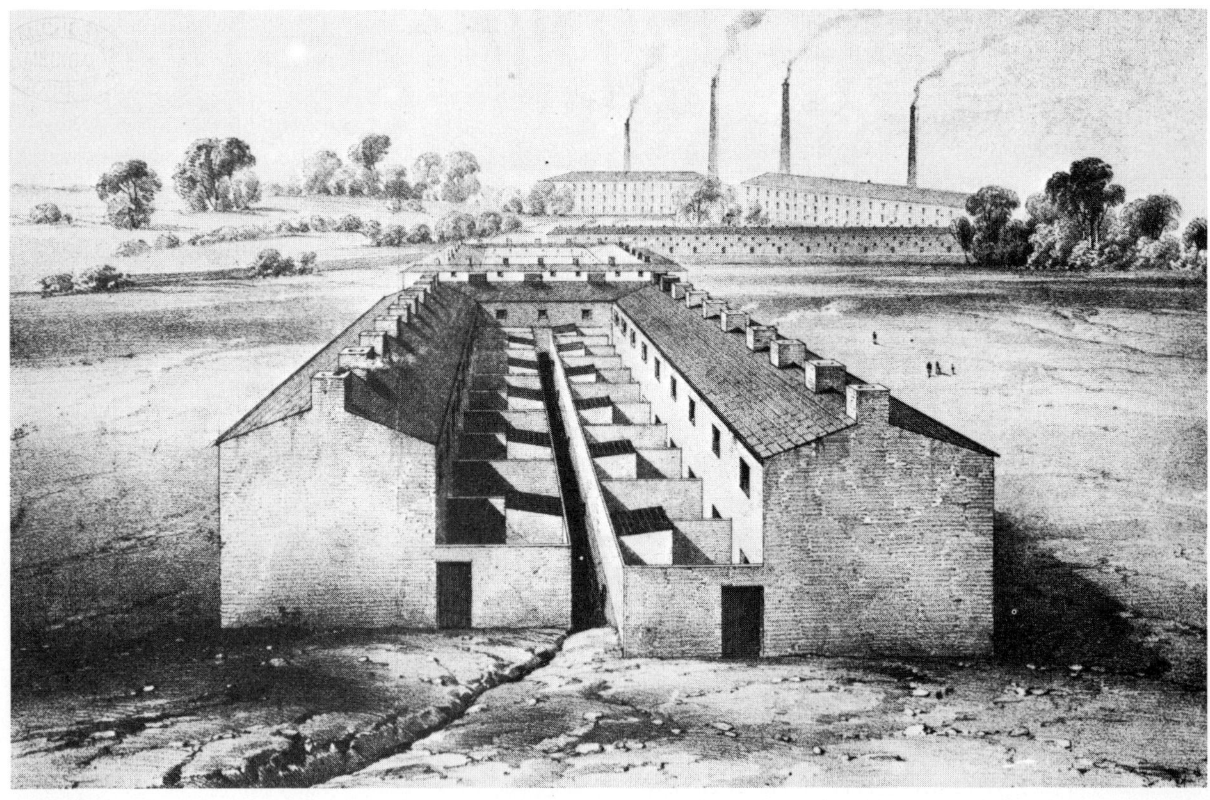

with its own tap and lavatory, in a properly drained street, for only $3\frac{1}{2}$d a week on the rent, far less than the cost of supporting families left destitute by disease. Chadwick included details and drawings of one of the most important, but least remembered, inventions of the nineteenth century — the narrow-bore, round, glazed earthenware drainpipe, which would carry sewage away far more efficiently than the old brick tunnels or wooden pipes. This was the key to his 'arterial system', under which every house would receive a piped water supply, the waste from which would carry away the household sewage.

The first Public Health Act

The *Report* created a sensation. Ten thousand copies were sold; it reached the Queen at Windsor Castle; it was used as a textbook in training engineers; it was quoted at public meetings all over the country; and it led to the setting up of a Royal Commission on the Health of Towns which discovered that out of fifty large towns only one had a satisfactory sewerage system and only six an adequate water supply. In 1844 the Health of Towns Association was formed to fight for sanitary reform, its keenest members being the doctors and clergy who had seen the effects of cholera

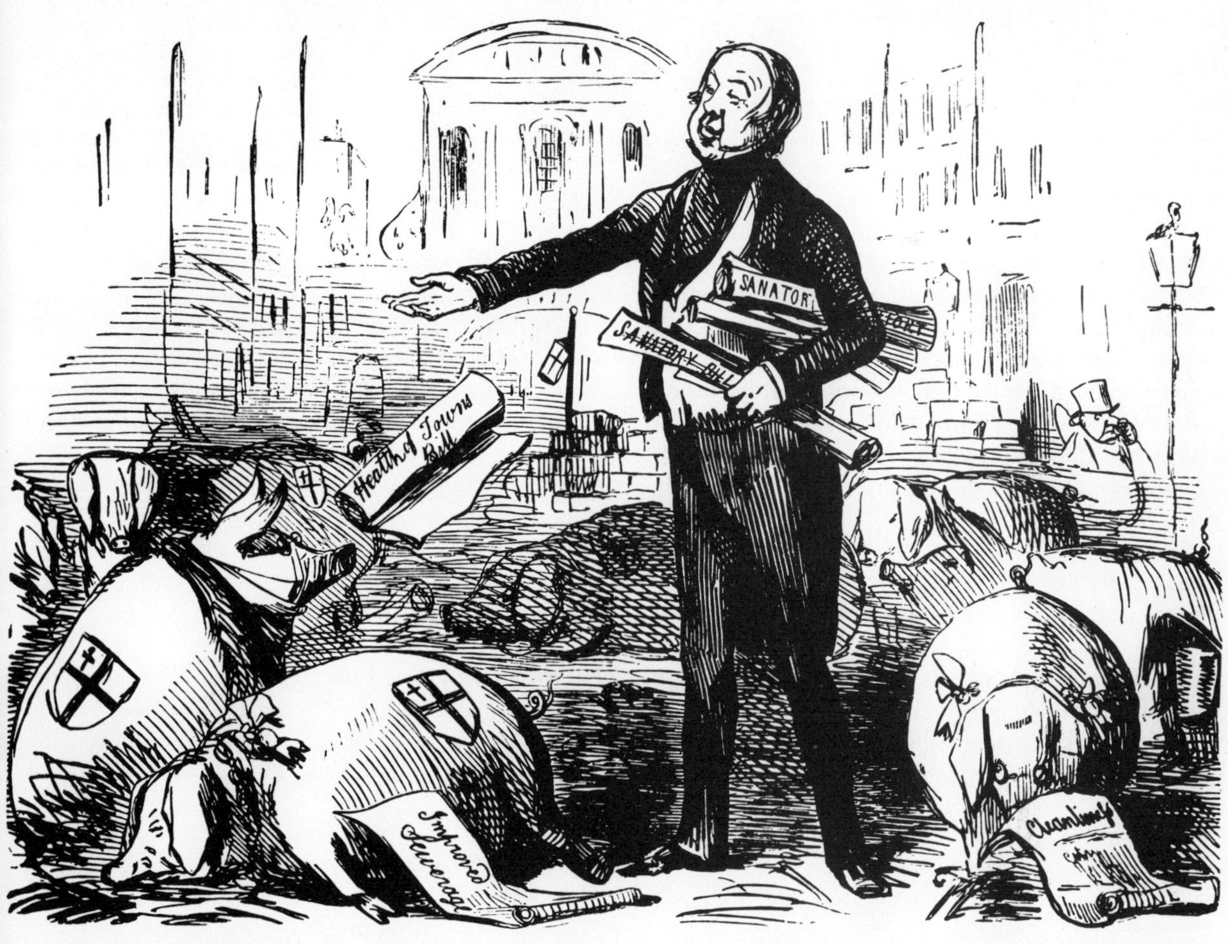

Lord Morpeth, the man who carried the first Public Health Act through parliament, as seen by *Punch*. The caption reads 'Lord Morpeth Throwing Pearls before – Aldermen'.

at first hand and had often served on local boards of health. Many M.P.s, however, were still unwilling to see the government accept responsibility for the public health. When, in 1847, a Public Health Bill was introduced into Parliament, it was dropped because of opposition from 'the dirty party' who disapproved of sanitary reform. It was only because the cholera was again approaching in 1848 – 'that appalling pest' one speaker called it, 'that dreadful scourge' another – that Parliament, terrified of another epidemic, carried the first Public Health Act. This incorporated Chadwick's idea 'that the supply of water . . . sewerage, drainage, cleansing and paving . . . should as far as practicable be under one and the same local management and control' and set up in London a national Board of Health for England and Wales. In all other towns either the corporation or, if the ratepayers chose, a specially elected local board of health, became officially responsible for carrying out the law, and especially unhealthy towns, with a death rate of more than twenty-three per 1,000, could be made to set up a board of health, whether they wanted to or not.

One of the members of the new central Board of

Health was Edwin Chadwick and another was the great philanthropist, Lord Ashley, better known as Lord Shaftesbury. The Board s Chief Medical Inspector was Dr Thomas Southwood Smith, who had worked with Chadwick on his East London inquiry and was Physician to the London Fever Hospital, 'fever' then meaning many infectious diseases, but especially typhus. Southwood Smith had originally trained as a nonconformist minister but abandoned it to become a doctor. He was a kindly man and while Chadwick was moved chiefly by the desire to save public money, Southwood Smith was inspired by sympathy for suffering.

The new Act came too late to save the country. Events in Merthyr Tydfil were typical. Years of neglect of this notoriously insanitary boom town led to a demand for a local board of health to be set up under the new law —but cholera appeared only a few weeks later and altogether 1,700 people died before it finally moved on. In the whole British Isles the cholera epidemic which swept the country between 1848 and 1849 killed about 130,000 people, while at least twice as many suffered from the disease. The old argument between contagionists and miasmatists remained unanswered, but the Board of Health favoured the miasmatists. Chadwick even declared, unscientifically, that 'All smell is disease'.

The Board of Health's energetic action made it very unpopular with many influential people. *The Times* declared that 'We prefer to take our chance of cholera and the rest than be bullied into health', and many M.P.s agreed. In 1854 the Board was overthrown, Chadwick, at fifty-three, and Southwood Smith, now aged sixty-six, being dismissed with a pension.

One mystery solved

While the Board of Health's inspectors had been hurrying about the country trying to fight one outbreak of cholera after another, a quiet, reserved London doctor had been exploring a theory of his own. John Snow had been born in York, the son of a farmer. After

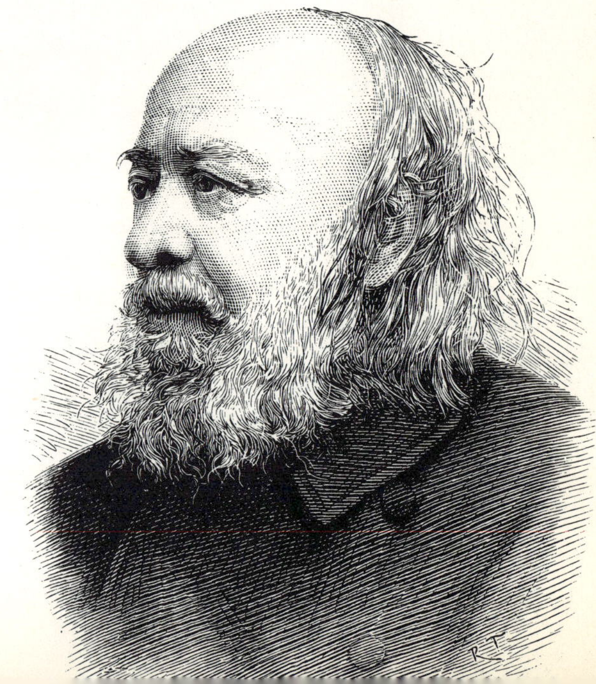

Edwin Chadwick, shown late in life, after he had received his well-earned knighthood. Unlike many later reformers (such as John Snow) Chadwick's reasons for promoting reform were not, first and foremost, humanitarian. Disease and ill-health were unpleasant, but more important they were *inefficient*. Children dying young could not work in factories; decrease in population meant less production; men who were often sick worked less well and less often. Strange though it seems now, we owe many of our most important reforms in the nineteenth century to this kind of argument.

being apprenticed to a surgeon in Newcastle he had, as a young medical student of eighteen, fought single handed a serious outbreak in a colliery village in 1831. Later he walked to London and set up in practice in Soho in central London.

Dr Snow was, for much of his life, a teetotaller and vegetarian and he never married. He was a generous man, always ready to visit a poor patient free, and invariably polite even to the least important person. As a researcher he was patient and systematic, rather than brilliant, but these are often the qualities that bring the best results. In 1849 he published a modestly-titled book, *On the Mode of Communication of Cholera*, which, for the first time, put forward the theory that cholera might be spread by the water supply. In 1854 there came the chance to test his ideas for there suddenly broke out in Soho what Dr Snow called 'the most terrible outbreak of cholera which ever occurred in this kingdom'. In two days 197 people died and in another week, in an area only 250 yards long, there were more than 500 deaths. If, reasoned John Snow, it was atmospheric conditions which caused the disease, why did it devastate one street but barely touch the next, since both breathed the same air? And why did nearly everyone in some houses catch cholera while people in the next door building escaped? Dr Snow soon discovered that the whole outbreak was centred on one pump, in Broad Street. 'The deaths,' he later wrote, 'either very much diminished, or ceased altogether, at every point where it becomes decidedly nearer to send to another pump than to the one in Broad Street.' In almost every house which had used the water the disease had appeared while not one of seventy men in a local brewery, who drank beer at work, caught it. Most conclusive of all, a woman in Hampstead, several miles away, and free of cholera, had formerly lived in Broad Street, and 'having developed a great taste

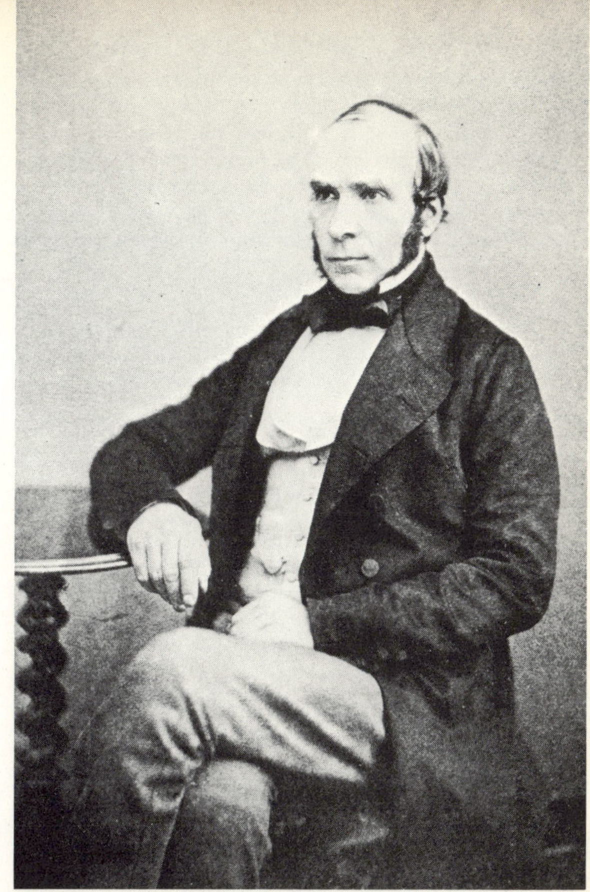

John Snow, aside from his work on public health and cholera, was also a pioneer of anaesthetics.

A pump in Fryingpan Alley, Clerkenwell.

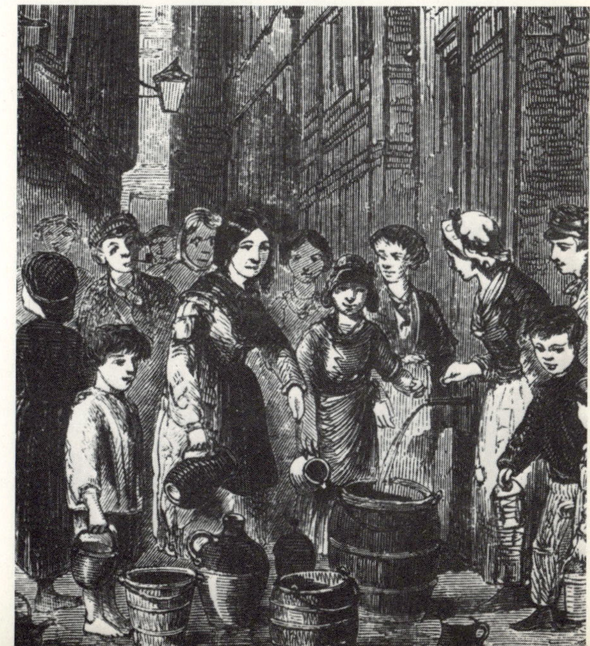

A re-drawn version of John Snow's map, showing deaths from cholera in the Broad Street area between 19 August and 30 September 1854. Snow was able to show that virtually all the victims had drunk from the pump in Broad Street, in spite of the fact that many of them lived some way away. The map also shows the brewery, which escaped untouched: the men working in the brewery drank beer.

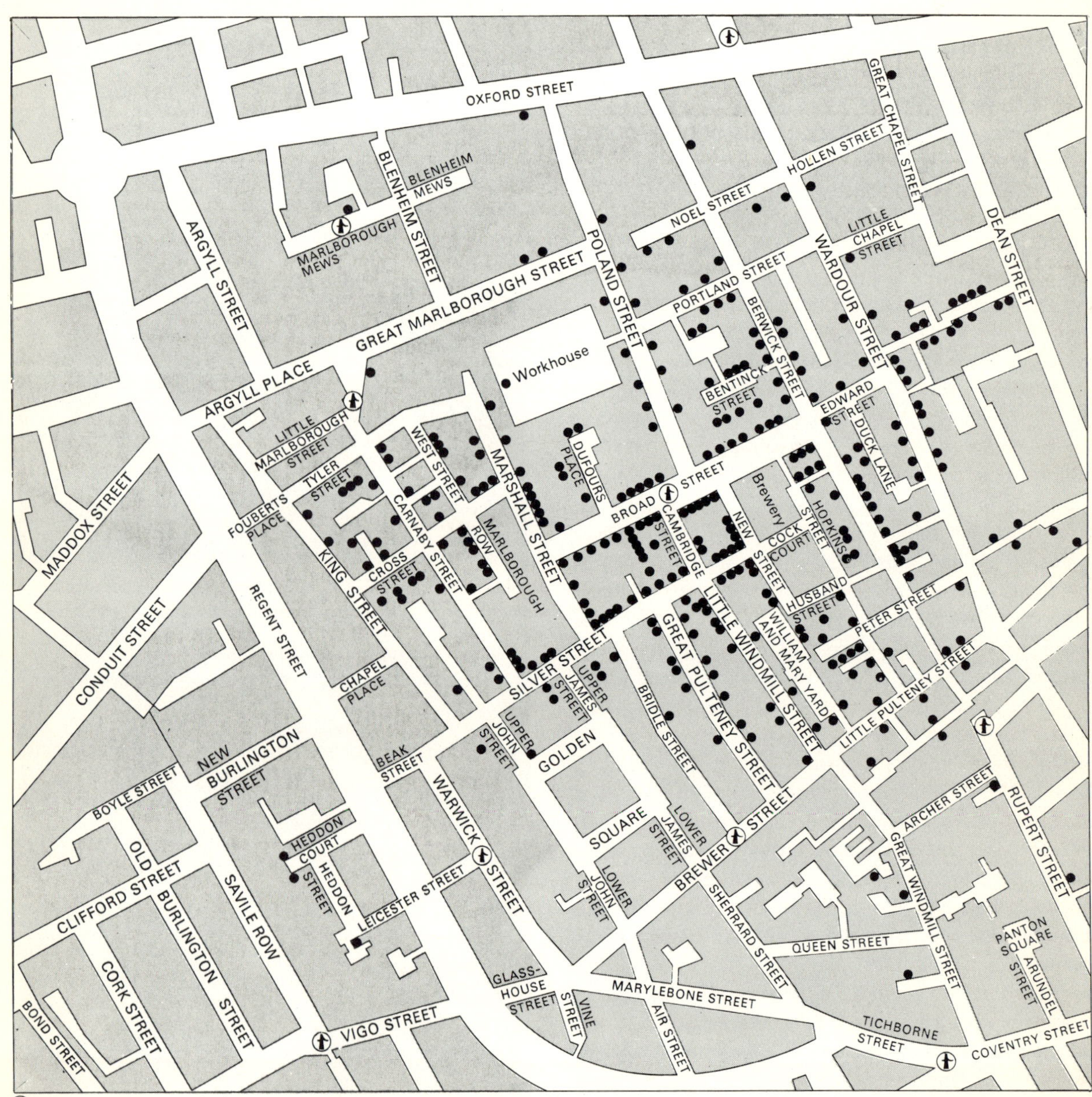

Pump   ● Deaths from cholera

One of the most important, but least noticed, figures in the history of public health was William Farr. Farr was a statistician – indeed some people would claim that he was the founder of the modern science of social statistics – and for most of his life he was responsible for the statistics that were compiled at the offices of the Registrar General. On one occasion in 1866 he noticed that the statistics of deaths from cholera appeared to be concentrated in one particular region of East London. Farr went to investigate. He found that the attacks coincided almost exactly with the area served by the East London Water Company, and in particular the Old Ford Reservoir. The company, of course, protested – but in a revealing way: one of the engineers innocently told Farr that there was nothing wrong with the water, 'he had eaten some excellent eels out of the Old Ford Reservoir'. One Alexander Russell of Paradise Cottages, Poplar, had another tale.

'A short time since, the water supply to my residence was stopped from what cause I could not imagine and I was without a supply five days. At length I took off the tap and to my astonishment found *an eel fourteen inches in length*. It was in a *putrid* state and the *stench* arising from it was most *fearful*. Since that time I have lost two of my children, who died of cholera, and my wife and other members of the family have also suffered from that disease.'

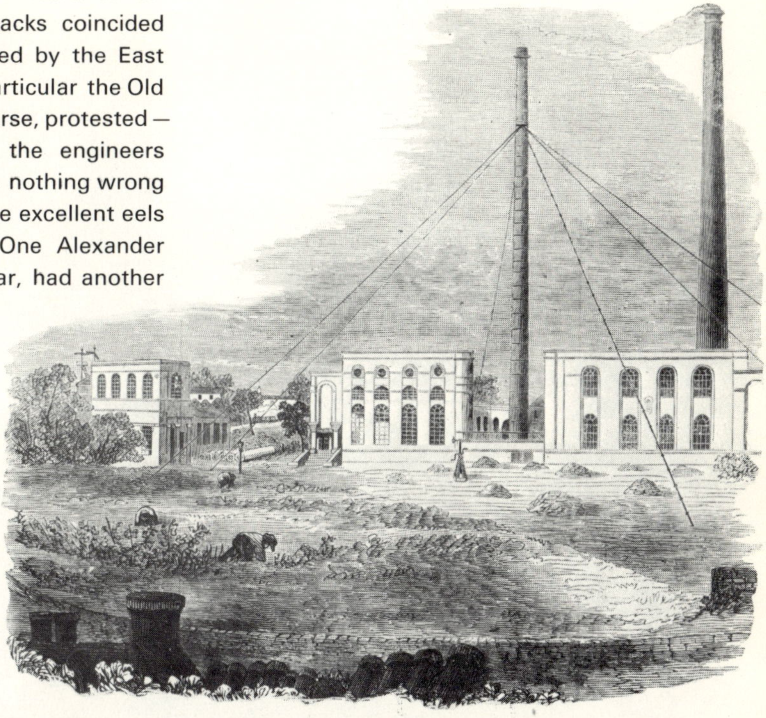

The Old Ford Reservoir of the East London Water Company.

for the Broad Street water, had a large bottle of it sent out on the carrier's cart every day to her new home'. One arrived on a Thursday; on Friday she was taken ill; on Saturday she died. Her niece, visiting her, drank some of the water, went home and died too – the only case in her district. Long before he discovered this, however, Dr Snow had persuaded the authorities to remove the handle of the Broad Street pump, thus forcing the local people to go elsewhere for their water. The results were immediate; the epidemic stopped as suddenly as it had begun.

Dr Snow was able to show, too, that piped water might be as dangerous as that from a pump if the original source were infected. By painstaking, door to door inquiries in an area of South London supplied by two different water companies, he proved that people whose water came originally from the sewage-ridden Thames at Battersea were fourteen times as likely to catch cholera as those who drank the purer water drawn off higher up-river. He even managed, by correspondence, to explain that disastrous outbreak two years before in the village of Newburn where, he

The Houses of Parliament themselves were notorious for bad air, and during the summer months members taking a stroll on the balcony needed a handkerchief to hold across their nose and mouth. The ventilation in the building was also very bad, and Henry Hunt, the radical leader, mildly pointed out that it was 'very stupid . . . to expose themselves to unnecessary danger while they were deliberating how they might best provide security for others'. *Punch* published this cartoon in 1858.

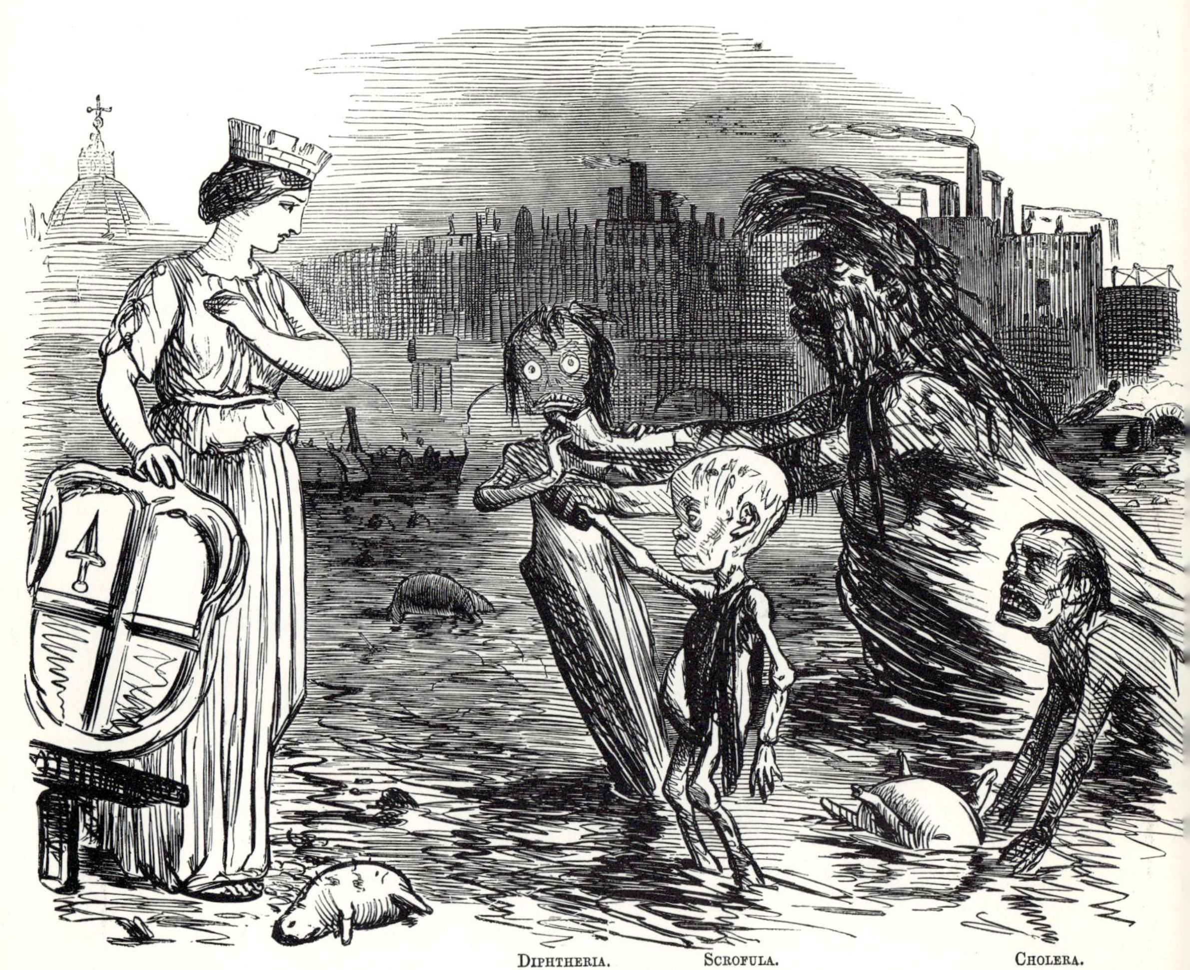

FATHER THAMES INTRODUCING HIS OFFSPRING TO THE FAIR CITY OF LONDO

(*A Design for a Fresco in the New Houses of Parliament.*)

The beginning of modern London, 1867, showing a cross-section of the Embankment, with the Metropolitan District Railway and the new sewerage system. Also included is a strange, forgotten piece of nineteenth-century engineering, marked 4 on the illustration. This was intended to be a tunnel for the 'Pneumatic Railway', a system which worked by propelling a carriage through a tube by means of compressed air.

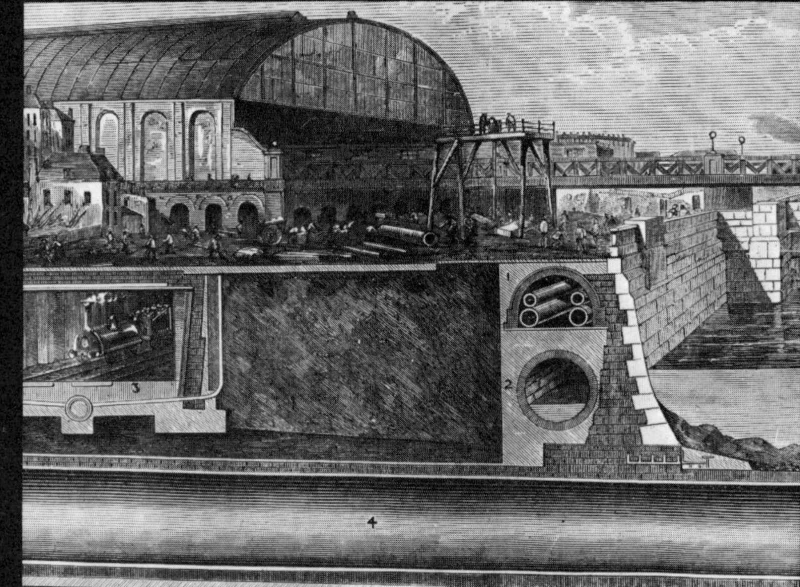

An advertisement for home water-filters in the 1870s.

SILICATED CARBON WATER-FILTERS.

THE MOST EFFECTIVE MEANS KNOWN OF PURIFYING WATER FOR DOMESTIC, MANUFACTURING, AND GENERAL PURPOSES.

These are the only Filters capable of thoroughly removing the organic and saline impurities, animalculæ, &c., from water. They are adopted, in preference to all others, by the Government, the authorities of the General Post Office, the London and Provincial Hospitals, and many other large public and private establishments in all parts of the world.

PRIZE MEDAL, PARIS EXHIBITION, 1867.

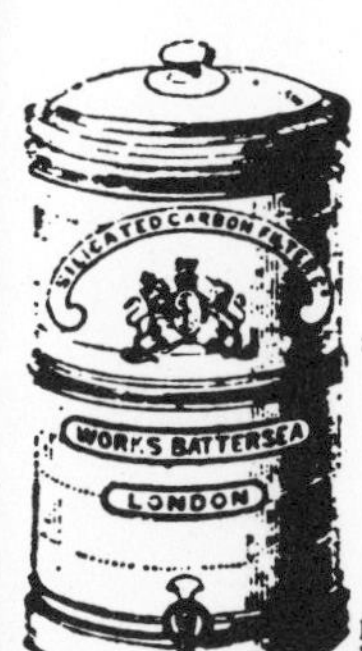

No. 27.

THE DOMESTIC FILTER.

No. 27.

Made in cream-coloured Stoneware, and fitted with slabs of Patent Silicated Carbon Filtering Media.

Complete with Cover and Plated Tap.

PRICES.

No. A,	capacity 1	gallon	14s. 6d.
No. B,	,, 2	,,	21s. 0d.
No. C,	,, 4	,,	33s. 0d.
No. D,	,, 6	,,	42s. 0d.
No. E,	,, 8	,,	52s. 0d.
No. F,	,, 12	,,	70s. 0d.

THE ONLY SILVER MEDAL, HAVRE EXHIBITION, 1868.

THE

DINING ROOM FILTER.

No. 22.

Made in marbled china, chaste and elegant in appearance, and well suited for the Dining-room.

Size A will purify six gallons per day; B, about twenty gallons; the water possessing that freshness which is always wanting in the ordinary Carbon Filters.

Prices, with Electro-Plated Tap, A, 30s.; B, 70s.

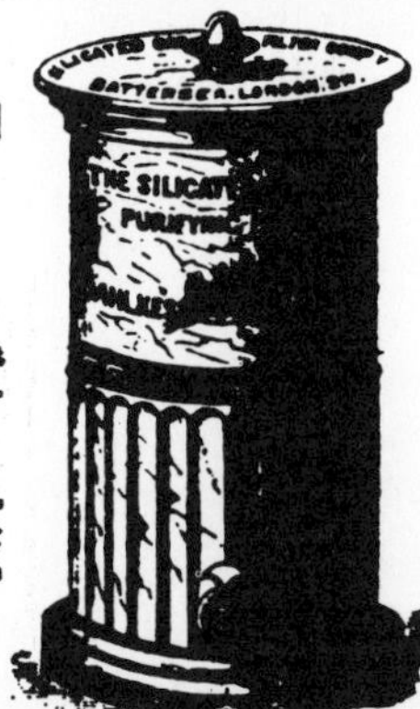

No. 22.

decided, it was not a pump or piped water but an infected stream that was to blame. He solved the mystery of why people living in crowded conditions so often caught cholera —they might touch each other's soiled bedding or clothes before eating their food. As for those strange cases where cholera seemed to leap across miles of countryside, Dr Snow had an answer to them, too. Perhaps, he suggested it was not infected air that was to blame, but infected flies, travelling through the air and depositing in hitherto harmless food and water the dirt they had picked up in cholera-stricken homes.

The end of the cholera story

We now know that John Snow was completely right in all his deductions and guesses, but when he published a new edition of his previous book, in 1855, it created little stir. He was even accused of holding back sanitary progress, because, it was argued, if the air was not to blame people would no longer bother about cleaning up 'nuisances' in the streets. Some doctors suggested that even if infected water did spread the disease it would only act on those already weakened by 'poisoned air'. Slowly, very slowly, everyone realized John Snow had been right and that cholera was mainly spread by the excrement of cholera patients getting into the water supply; the air had nothing whatever to do with it. But getting rid of a false theory, once it is firmly lodged, takes a long time. There were still some miasmatists at large in England nearly half a century later and some were active in Germany right into the present century.

John Snow himself did not live to see the final vindication of his theory, for he died of a stroke in 1858 at the age of forty-four while hard at work on a new subject, the relief of pain. Eight years after his death, in 1866, the last great cholera epidemic in the British Isles provided conclusive proof of his theory, when 7,000 people in the East End of London died of cholera in a few weeks, after a new employee at a waterworks had allowed unfiltered water, containing sewage from a house where cholera was present, to enter the main water supply.

The lesson was not forgotten. Soon, with sanitary conditions tremendously improved and a pure water supply, cholera in the British Isles belonged to the past. A few small outbreaks in 1892 and 1893 never developed into serious epidemics; in the worst only thirty people died. The very last person to die of cholera on British soil was a foreign seaman, who had picked up the disease abroad — and even that was sixty years ago. Today cholera is only a problem in countries with low standards of hygiene and sanitation. In 1947, for instance, 10,000 people died of cholera in Egypt, and every year about the same number die of it in India and Pakistan, the real homes of the disease. Doctors believe, however, that with improved conditions it can be stamped out even there and become a mere memory, like the Black Death.

The development of public health

Impressive public health measures were taken in Ancient Rome: the main sewerage system was in operation as early as the sixth century B.C. Later, aqueducts were built to supply the city with fresh water, and public baths were provided not only in Rome, but also in outposts of the Empire. In Britain, remains of Roman baths can still be seen in places such as Bath and Wroxeter.

1816 A children's dispensary founded in London and 'visitors' organized to educate mothers in child care.

1833 Lord Shaftesbury's first Factory Act limited the working day of children under the age of eleven to nine hours and, for those between the ages of eleven and eighteen, to twelve hours. Government inspectors were appointed to see that this was carried out.

1837 Registration of births, marriages and deaths made obligatory in Britain. This helped to provide statistics on disease because the cause of death had to be given.

1839 Meeting in Constantinople between Turkey and various foreign powers on the question of quarantine. A number of regulations were laid down, but the atmosphere was embittered by trade rivalries.

1842 Chadwick's report, *The Sanitary Condition of the Labouring Population*, published.

1847 Britain's first Medical Officer of Health appointed in Liverpool.

1848 The first Public Health Act set up a national Board of Health in London and local boards in other towns.

1854 (31 July) The fall of the first Board of Health and the dismissal of Chadwick and Southwood Smith. (31 August) The second Board of Health set up with a remodelled policy.

1858 Abolition of the second Board of Health. Responsibility for public health passed to the Privy Council and, in 1871, to the Local Government Board. Vaccination against smallpox made compulsory in Britain.

1862 The Peabody Trust established. It attracted large donations for the poor of London. The establishment of the Trust was followed by what became known as '5 per cent philanthropy', in which people with capital could both improve the housing conditions of the poor *and* make a reasonable profit.

1864 The Factory Act in this year was the first of a series of acts on industrial problems such as lead-poisoning, ventilation and sanitation.

1866 Sanitary Act made inspectors compulsory for city areas.

1866–7 Labourers Dwellings Act made public money available for the building of labourers' houses.

1875 The Public Health Act in this year forced local authorities to install adequate drainage and sewerage systems in their towns and an adequate water supply. Ratepayers' money could, for the first time, be spent on providing other amenities such as parks, hospitals and public lavatories.
Artisans and Labourers Dwellings Improvement Act allowed local authorities to rebuild slum areas and to build and let their own houses. This was the beginning of council houses as we know them today, but little was actually done as a result of this law, partly because the cost of compensation for compulsory purchase was too high. This law was strengthened by succeeding Acts in 1890 and 1919.

1881 The spread of typhoid, scarlet fever and diptheria epidemics found to be caused by infected milk. Pasteurization of milk soon followed.

1888 Parliament created county councils and boroughs which became vital in the carrying out of new laws on public health.

1892 A pioneer system of child welfare clinics set up in France and widely copied in Europe.

1906 Education (Provision of Meals) Act enabled local authorities to provide meals in school for children from poor families. Progressive authorities, such as London, Manchester and Liverpool, extended schemes already in operation.

1907 Medical Department created at the Board of Education. It encouraged local education authorities to give medical inspections to children in elementary schools and, in 1918, an Education Act obliged them to provide treatment for any physical or mental defects discovered during these inspections.

1919 Ministry of Health created.

1923 League of Nations created a Health Organization which produced reports on public health topics.

1934 Public funds first used to provide milk in schools at a low price.

1946 World Health Organization took over the duties and powers of the League of Nations' Health Organization. Amongst a wide range of work, it helps to control the spread of epidemics.

1948 National Health Service introduced in Britain.

4 The doctor and the patient

The status of the doctor

Today the doctor holds such a recognized place in society that it is hard to realize that medicine was once a far less respected profession than many others. Nowadays doctors are recognized as people of some standing in the community, and are entitled to expect a reasonable living in return for their highly responsible job. An average general practitioner in the Health Service, for example, earns at least £4,000 a year and a top-class consultant in a hospital may earn up to £10,000. To become qualified a doctor has to measure up to a high educational and intellectual standard and to survive six years of rigorous training, with at least a year's experience working under supervision in a hospital. The family doctor himself commands a wide range of means of diagnosis and treatment, but can always refer a patient to an even more highly qualified and better equipped specialist, who may have devoted almost his whole working life to studying a particular problem. Doctors, like people in other occupations, vary widely in ability, but anyone consulting a British-trained doctor knows he must, at least at some time in his life, have fulfilled certain minimum requirements of skill and knowledge.

In the 1830s none of these conditions applied. Many doctors had never passed an examination in their lives and had done their training at small medical schools run by badly qualified people for private profit. Only since 1815 has anyone entering the profession been required by law to follow a recognized course of study and serve a five-year apprenticeship giving him practical experience, and it was not till 1858 that Parliament passed the Medical Registration Act setting up a General Register of the whole profession, supervised by the General Medical Council. The Council prevented anyone who was not properly qualified being admitted to the Register and could 'strike off' anyone guilty of unprofessional conduct.

Twenty pounds a year

Up to this time the medical profession was really divided into three, with great social distinctions between them —the first *Medical Directory* to include all types of doctors did not appear until 1845. The recognized leaders of the medical profession were the physicians, men who had a medical degree, belonged to one of the exclusive national Colleges of Physicians, and usually practised among better-off people or were called in as consultants. The ordinary general practitioner was usually an apothecary, the old name for a chemist. The early nineteenth-century apothecary often made up and sold his own medicine over the counter of his own shop, and also visited patients in their homes. His training was usually sketchy and he

An engraving of an eighteenth-century apothecary.

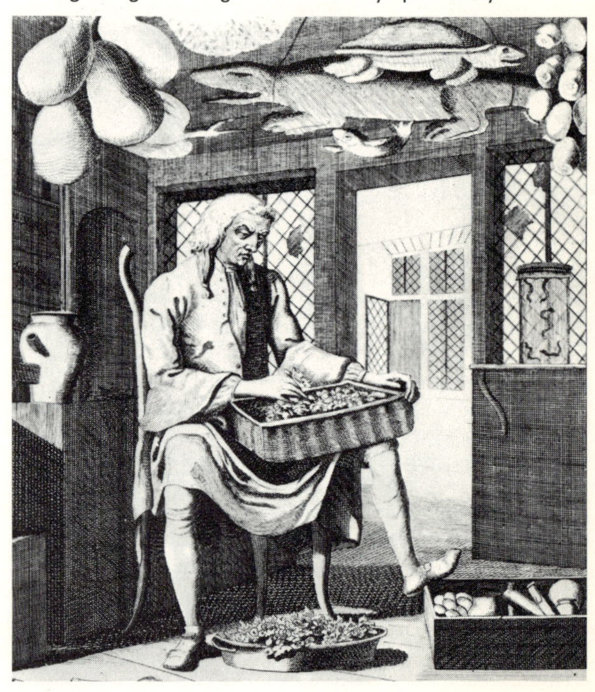

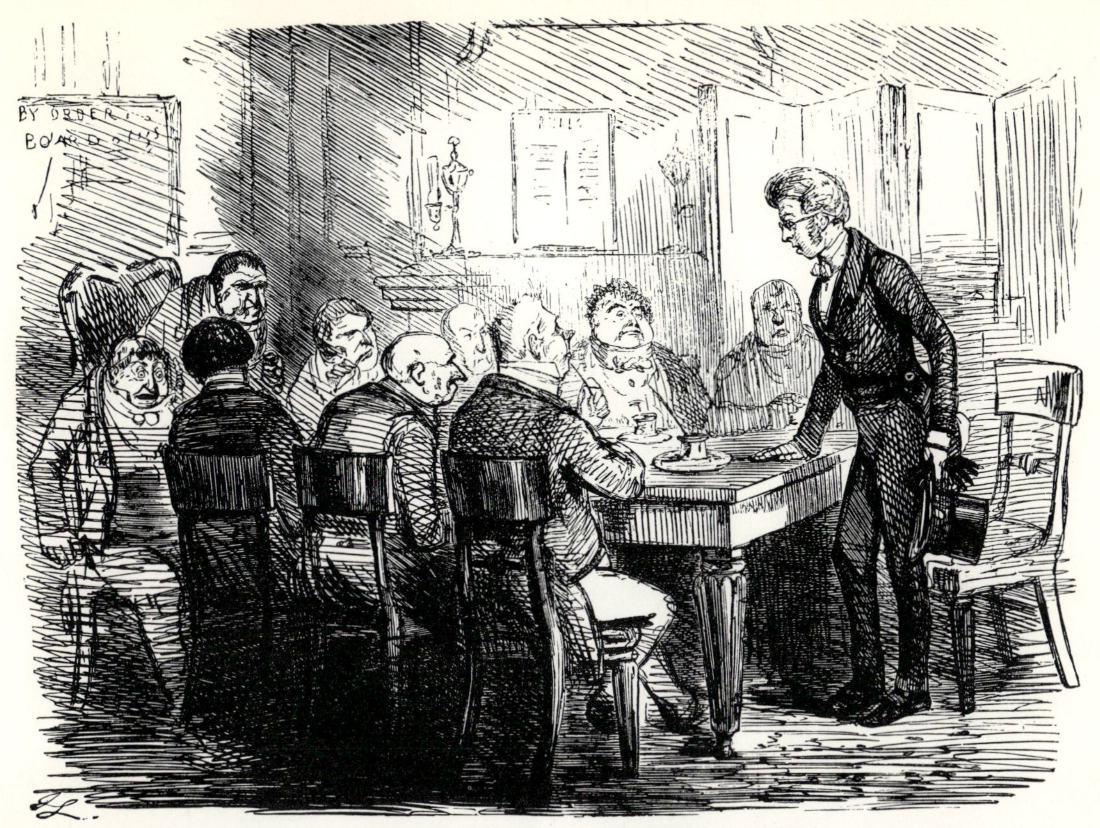

SPLENDID OPENING FOR A YOUNG MEDICAL MAN.

Chairman. "Well, young man. So you wish to be engaged as Parish Doctor?"
Doctor. "Yes, Gentlemen, I am desirous——"
Chairman. "Ah! Exactly. Well—It's understood that your wages—salary I should say—is to be twenty pounds per annum; and you find your own tea and sugar—medicines I mean—and, in fact, make yourself generally useful. If you do your duty, and conduct yourself properly, why—ah—you—ah——"
[*Punch.* "Will probably be bowled out of your situation by some humbug, who will fill it for less money."]

measured his earnings in shillings rather than pounds. Even if he had a regular income from a friendly society for attending its members, or from a parish or Board of Guardians (who were responsible for caring for the destitute poor of the district), this was probably very small. For working day and night for weeks in the great cholera epidemics, many parish doctors received no extra pay and some were even required to pay for all the medicines they prescribed out of their own pocket. When they complained they were told by unsympathetic local officials that they had no more right to extra money than a painter who had quoted too low an estimate for a job —the point being that the doctor was regarded by middle-class people as a tradesman, not as a privileged member of a learned profession.

Their own physicians the wealthy might treat with more respect — but not much more. There is a case on record of a sick countess who sent her maid to describe her symptoms to the doctor as she would not lower herself to speak to him in person. The cartoon from *Punch* in 1848 on this page shows a committee interviewing a candidate for the job of parish doctor. 'Well,' the chairman is saying, 'it's understood that your wages — salary, I should say — is to be twenty pounds per annum; and you find your own tea and sugar — medicines I mean — and in fact, make yourself generally useful . . . and conduct yourself properly.' In other words, the doctor was being spoken to exactly as if he were applying for a job as a domestic servant.

Left A nurse in the late eighteenth century, as seen by Thomas Rowlandson. *Centre* Florence Nightingale, described as 'An Angel of Mercy'. Her work in the Crimean War did a great deal to enhance the status of nurses, and indeed of women in general. Yet here the nurse is seen not really as a professional medical person, but as a substitute for a devoted mother, wife or daughter. *Right* The new style, of 1916: trained and efficient, if a little starched.

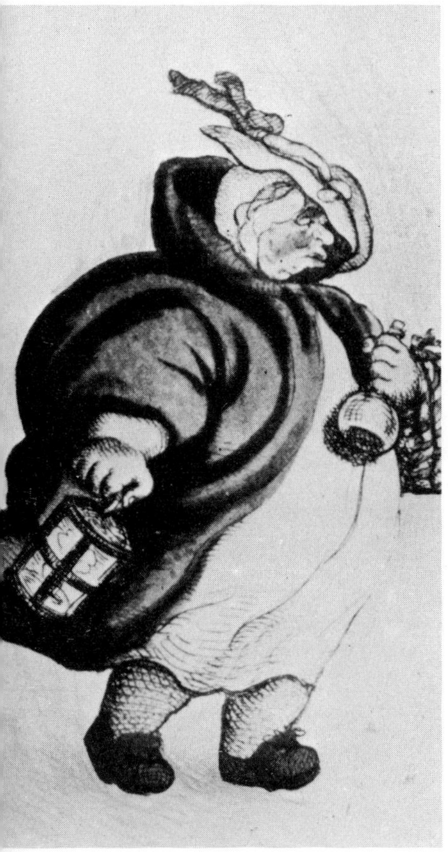

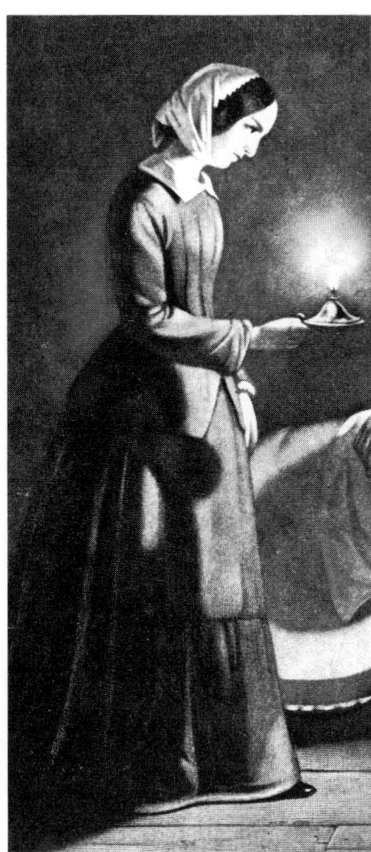

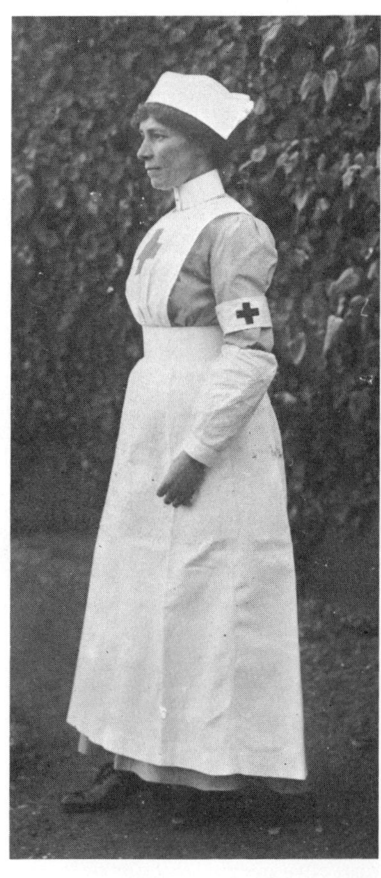

Nurses

Nursing was also regarded as an inferior profession. For generations it had been seen as a job for the lowest type of uneducated and unintelligent women, often elderly widows. Night nurses were sometimes known as 'watchers' since all they did was keep an eye on the patient and most of the great hospitals have cases in their records like that of Guy's Hospital in 1859, where the Matron recorded: 'It has been necessary in Stephen Ward to dismiss three out of four women employed . . . and last night the nurse of Petersham Ward was completely incapacitated for work on account of drink.' Until about this time nurses spent much of their time scrubbing the floors and had no uniform, being regarded as another kind of char-woman. A matron who succeeded in recruiting nurses who were actually sober, did not steal from the patient and had enough education to read the label on a bottle of medicine, thought herself very lucky indeed.

An amputation as seen by Thomas Rowlandson in 1785.

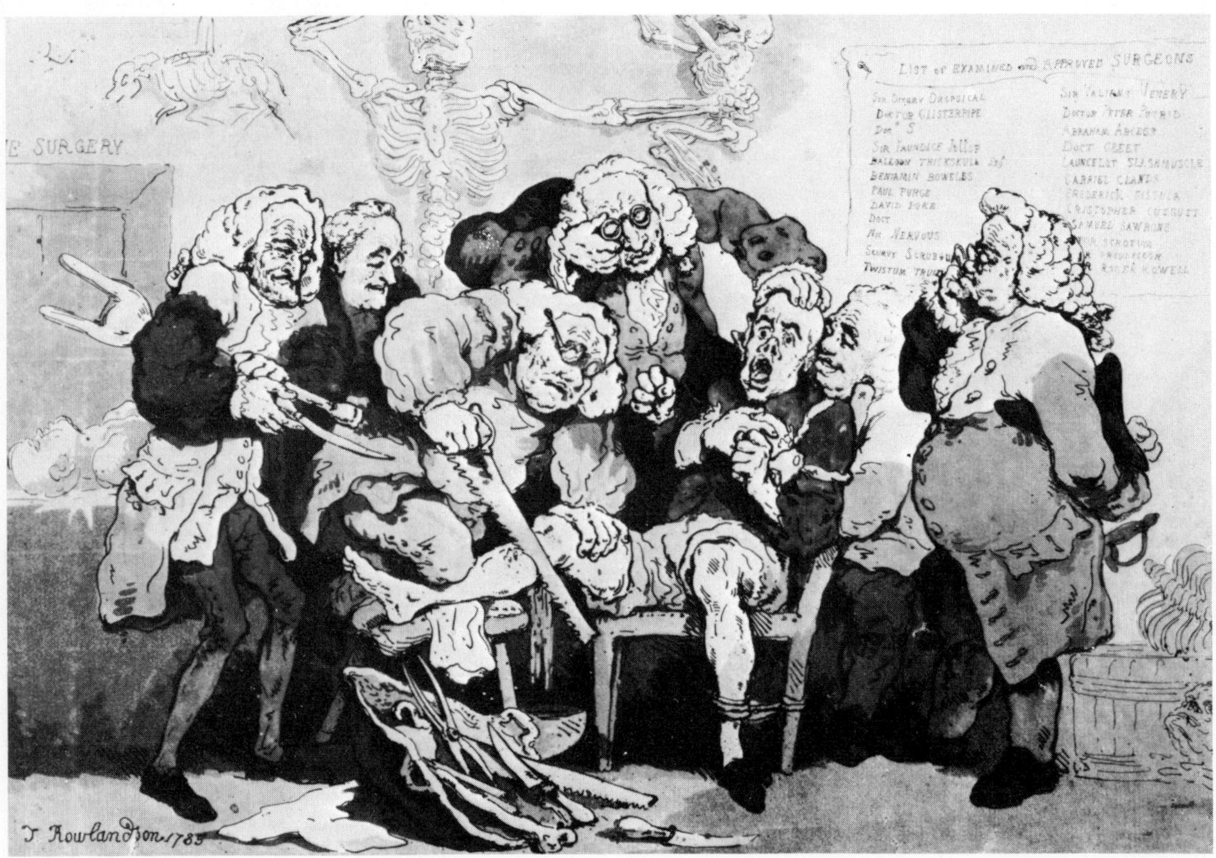

From sawbones to surgeon

But the most despised section of the whole medical profession were the surgeons – apart, that is, from a few eminent men working in a few famous hospitals. Often they were ill-trained, since, as has been mentioned, there was a grave shortage of bodies for dissection and an aura of horror surrounded the whole subject of anatomy in the public mind. Their field of work was in any case extremely limited, since with no means of putting the patient to sleep and no way of protecting him from infection after an operation, few operations were attempted and even those few were often fatal. The commonest operations up to about 1850 were amputations, removal of stone in the bladder, the excision of tumours and the treatment of swollen arteries. It was not surprising that the surgeon was often looked down on as a mere 'sawbones', only turned to as a last resort. The arrival of the physician meant, one hoped, recovery; the coming of the surgeon meant probable death.

The status of the medical profession

Public medical officers were often an essential part of society in Ancient Greece. They were the best known of public experts and often worked closely with architects on such projects as drainage and water supply.

In the Roman Empire there were valuable privileges for physicians. Julius Caesar, for example, gave Roman citizenship to physicians from Greece and elsewhere and, later, the Emperor Augustus freed all physicians from taxes.

1421 The Privy Council given authority to restrict medical practice to adequately trained physicians and surgeons, but these powers were not used.

1512 A Medical Act restricted practice to graduates of the two universities, Oxford and Cambridge, and to others licensed by the bishop of their diocese.

1518 Royal College of Physicians established.

1523 The College given the power to examine anyone wishing to practise medicine.

1540 The College allowed to examine apothecaries' shops and to test their drugs.
Act of Parliament united the Company of Barbers with the Company of Surgeons and allowed them the bodies of four executed criminals each year for dissecting purposes.

1617 Society of Apothecaries founded. From then on, apothecaries became the mainstay of general practice.

1703 As a result of a legal battle between the Royal College of Physicians and an apothecary, all apothecaries were legally allowed to treat the sick and prescribe drugs, but not to charge for visiting.

1800 Royal College of Surgeons formed. Its diploma carried with it the right to practise surgery.

1815 Apothecaries Act set up examinations by the Society of Apothecaries. No apothecary could practise without this qualification or a five-year apprenticeship.

1832 Anatomy Act allowed medical schools to obtain corpses for dissection by students. This greatly improved medical education.

1854 Florence Nightingale revolutionized nursing by her work at Scutari during the Crimean War.

1857 College of Dentists founded.

1859 First official list of qualified medical practitioners, the Medical Register, set up following the Medical Registration Act of 1858.

1859 First licences issued to dentists by the Royal College of Surgeons making dentistry a separate branch of the profession.

1860 Nightingale Training School for Nurses formed at St Thomas's Hospital by public subscription in response to Florence Nightingale's campaign for reform.

1865 Elizabeth Garrett Anderson, the first woman to qualify as a doctor in Britain, struggled hard to get into medical school: first at the Middlesex Hospital in London, then at St Andrews in Scotland and finally at Edinburgh. Each time she met prejudice among teachers, students and hospital staff. The men thought women were incapable of intense study without damage to their systems, and the women believed that a woman's place was in the home. Even after attending special courses at all three medical schools mentioned, together with a further course at the London Hospital and private tuition, no medical school would allow her to take an examination. So she turned to the Society of Apothecaries and, by threatening them with legal action, she was able to take the necessary qualifying examinations. She passed. This was in 1865 and, in the following year, she was admitted to the Medical Register, though it was another twelve years before any other women joined her.

1867 Metropolitan Poor Act began a series of new London infirmaries for the poor where probationary nurses were accepted for training.

1892 Three years' training for nurses recommended, but not enforced.

1902 Midwives Act established a register and training schools. Up until this time, district nursing societies usually employed 'cottage' or 'village' nurses for maternity cases. Some had a brief practical training, but most were untrained and uneducated.

1916 Royal College of Nursing founded.

1919 Nurses Registration Act set up nationally recognized examinations and a State Register.

1943 Nurses Act established two grades: the State Registered Nurse with a minimum of three years' training, and the Assistant Nurse with two years' training.

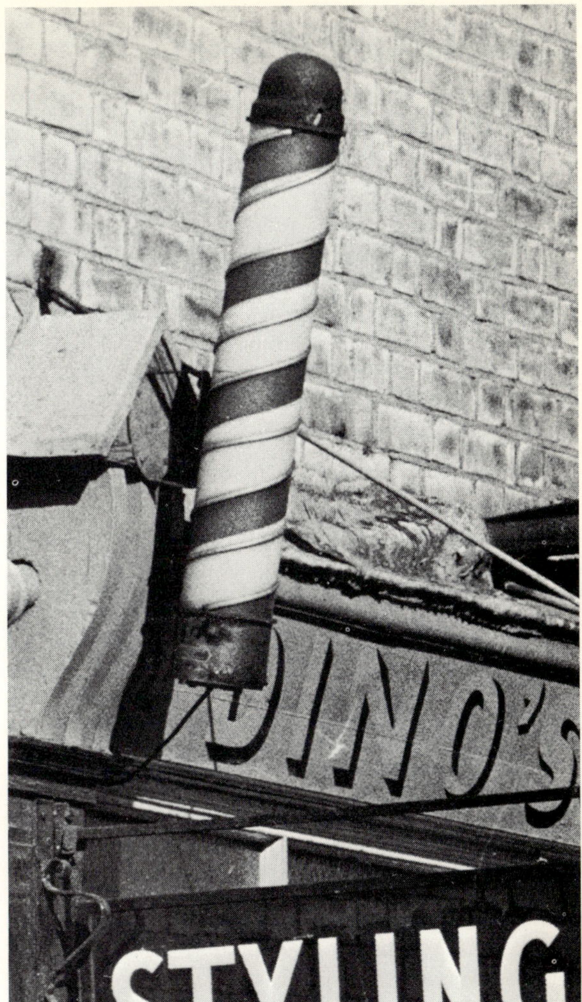

The barber's pole is still a familiar sight, but what it stood for has long been forgotten. Originally the sign indicated that surgery was practised, and the red and white stripes symbolized bandages over an injured limb.

The cruel knife

It also meant excruciating agony. Today no one would dream of even a minor operation, like having a tooth extracted, without at least a local anaesthetic to kill the pain, but until the middle of the nineteenth century there was no reliable way of making the body insensitive to pain, or rendering a patient unconscious. One doctor who had himself suffered at the surgeon's hands described his feelings in 1848 in a letter to another doctor:

> Before the days of anaesthetics a patient preparing for an operation was like a condemned criminal preparing for execution. He counted the days till the appointed day came. He counted the hours of that day till the appointed hour came. He listened for the echo in the street of the surgeon's carriage. He watched for his pull at the door bell, for his foot on the stair, for his step in the room, for the production of his dreaded instruments . . . and then he surrendered his liberty and . . . submitted to be held or bound, and helplessly gave himself up to the cruel knife.

Only the most ruthless surgeon could stay unmoved as the patient's screams rang in his ears and he struggled to get free. It was said of two famous surgeons that they could never 'think of an operation without heart sickness' and of another that he 'turned pale as death' whenever he performed one. There are horrifying descriptions on record of patients struggling desperately to escape in mid-operation from the attendants who held them, or dragging themselves back in terror across the floor, while the surgeon pursued them to finish his work. Sometimes the remarkable courage of the victim earned a round of applause from the medical students who crowded the operating theatre to watch, but usually an operation was a revolting experience for participants and observers alike. At this time everyone knew that the only answer to the patient's sufferings was greater and greater speed, even though this increased the risk of a mistake. By the careful standards of today the speed of operations was almost unbelievable. One man removed a stone from the bladder in fifty-four seconds; an arm or leg might be cut off in a minute or less. Once an American doctor crossed the Atlantic especially to see a famous British surgeon at work, but at the vital moment of the first incision he turned away to sneeze. When he looked back the operation was already over. Many doctors invited their students to time them and in a foreign hospital one callous surgeon actually placed a bet that he could remove a woman's breast in record time. He won his bet, but the patient died.

5 The hospital and the patient

Although Florence Nightingale's work in founding the profession of nursing is still remembered, it is often forgotten that she was also active in reforming hospital conditions in other directions, for example in improving hospital design and ventilation, cleanliness and diet. There was much to be done. The Royal Northern Hospital had no bath at all until 1860 and even then it had only cold water laid on. As late as 1874 the Westminster Hospital had only two fixed baths and one on wheels, to be shared between all the wards.

Even after the need for greater cleanliness had been recognized, a hospital remained a very dangerous place which you hardly expected to leave alive. Until well into the nineteenth century one famous London hospital, 'Bart's' (St Bartholomew's) asked for a deposit of 19s 6d before admitting patients, to pay their burial expenses if they died, and a doctor who recommended that a child should go into hospital might be asked, 'But who is going to pay for the funeral?' In her *Notes on Hospitals*, Florence Nightingale revealed that of nearly 13,000 people admitted to the 106 chief hospitals in England in 1861, more than 7,000 – 57 per cent – died, and in twenty-four London hospitals the rate was actually more than 90 per cent. 'Facts such as these', she commented, 'have sometimes raised grave doubts as to the advantages to be derived from hospitals at all and have led many to think that in all probability a poor sufferer would have a much better chance of recovery if treated at home.'

One reason for the appalling death rate was that because hospitals *were* so unhealthy, patients only entered them as a last resort, when desperately ill. But another reason worried the medical profession even more – that most of the deaths were due to diseases caught in hospital. As medical (or non-surgical) and surgical cases were commonly put in the same wards, until nearly the end of the nineteenth century, an infectious disease might spread from the former to the latter. One disease, typhus, was so common in hospitals that it was known as 'hospital fever', which began as an ache in the head, back and limbs, followed by mulberry-like spots all over the body, and ended in collapse, heart failure or pneumonia.

But the patient died

Of all those admitted to hospital, however, the patients in the greatest peril were surgical cases. Over and over again the surgeons recorded in their notes the classic obituary, 'The operation was successful but the patient died.' Sir James Simpson, who discovered chloroform, considered that 'The man laid on an operating table in one of our surgical hospitals is exposed to more chances of death than was the English soldier on the field of Waterloo. . . . A patient was safer in the gutter than in a hospital.'

This was an exaggeration, but only just. After one of the commonest forms of operation, amputation, 40 per cent of the patients in the great Scottish infirmaries of Edinburgh and Glasgow died. University College Hospital, London, was proud of its 'successful' record: a death rate after amputations of only one patient in four. The natural consequence of such experience was that operations were a rarity. Today some two million are carried out each year in National Health Service Hospitals in England and Wales and a large hospital has several operating theatres, which are used at all times of the day and night, seven days a week. In the 1860s and earlier an operation was such an unusual event that a notice saying 'Operation Today' would be posted to warn the students not to miss it and a bell would be rung as a reminder just before it started. An audience of hundreds might crowd into the gallery of the operating theatre itself to watch the surgeons at work, shouting, fighting and kicking down the dust from the wooden floors on to

In war poor medical facilities and sanitary conditions had, if anything, more serious effects than in the industrial towns. At least one historian has estimated that the Russo-Japanese War of 1904–5 was the first war in his history in which more people died in battle than from disease.

William Howard Russell was a talented Irishman who reported the entire Crimean War for *The Times*. His reports did a great deal to arouse the public's anger about the incompetence of the way the war was handled and the appalling conditions of the troops, including the hospitals. Below, a picture of Florence Nightingale's new style hospital.

The French losses from cholera were frightful. Convinced that there was something radically wrong in the air of the hospital at Varna, the French cleared out of the building altogether, and resolved to treat their cases in the field. The hospital had been formerly used as a Turkish barrack. It was a huge quadrangular building, like the barracks at Scutari, with a courtyard in the centre. The sides of the square were about 150 feet long, and each of them contained three floors, consisting of spacious corridors, with numerous rooms off them of fair height and good proportions. About one-third of the building was reserved for our use; the remainder was occupied by the French. Although not very old, the building was far from being in thorough repair. The windows were broken, the walls in parts were cracked and shaky, and the floors were mouldering and rotten. Like all places which have been inhabited by Turkish soldiers for any time, the smell of the buildings was abominable. Men sent in there with fevers and other disorders were frequently attacked with the cholera in its worst form and died with unusual rapidity, in spite of all that could be done to save them. I visited the hospital and observed that a long train of carts filled with sick soldiers were drawn up by the walls. There were thirty-five carts, with three or four men in each. These were sick French soldiers sent in from the camps and waiting till room could be found for them in the hospital. A number of soldiers were sitting down by the roadside and here and there the moonbeams flashed brightly off their piled arms. The men were silent; not a song, not a laugh. A gloom, seldom seen among French troops, reigned amid these groups of grey-coated men and the quiet that prevailed was only broken now and then by the moans and cries of the poor sufferers in the carts. Observing that about fifteen arabas without any occupants were waiting in the square, I asked a *sous-officier* for what purpose they were required. His answer, sullen and short, was – 'Pour les morts – pour les Français décédés, Monsieur.'

William Howard Russell

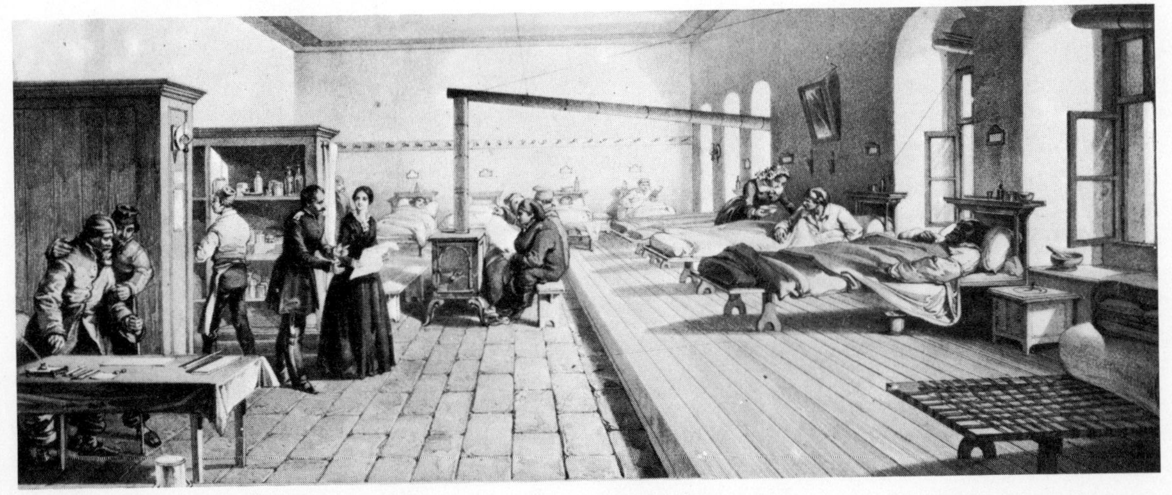

the operating table. In the whole of 1868 in one of the largest and most famous hospitals in the country, Guy's, there were only 364 major operations — and that was the greatest number for years. The results were not very encouraging. All three double amputations had proved fatal, both Caesarean operations and the only attempt to remove the spleen. Of the more routine operations, three of the fourteen men operated on for hernia had died, five of the sixteen women who had had gynaecological operations, and four of the thirteen cases of tracheotomy, which involved cutting open the windpipe. Altogether sixty-seven surgical patients had died — a remarkably low death rate for the time. In 1967 in Guy's Hospital, 13,200 operations were performed; the number of deaths was extremely small.

The conquest of pain

Two things were to change all this. The first was the conquest of pain. In 1839 a great French surgeon declared positively that 'The avoidance of pain while operating is an idea for a fairy tale and we should not concern ourselves with it any more. The cutting of the knife and pain are two aspects of surgery which cannot be separated.' Within only a few years he had to admit himself wrong.

It is hard to say who actually discovered anaesthetics, for several men, on both sides of the Atlantic, had the basic idea while others developed it for practical use. The real pioneers were two American dentists, who used 'laughing gas' (nitrous oxide) and ether respectively when extracting teeth. The first major operation carried out under ether in England was performed at University College Hospital, London, in December 1846 by Robert Liston, a leading surgeon who, it was said, could amputate a thigh 'in as few seconds as a first-class sprinter takes to run a hundred yards'. The first anaesthetized patient was a thirty-six year old butler. The last words he heard were Liston saying, 'Gentlemen, we are now going to try a Yankee dodge for making men insensible.' Twenty-six seconds after Liston had begun the operation the patient's diseased leg lay on the floor — and its owner had clearly felt nothing and had slept soundly.

In the following year there was another famous scene, in the dining room of an Edinburgh doctor, James Simpson, who, as a student, had seen Robert Liston operate on a Highland woman without an anaesthetic and had never forgotten her sufferings. After using ether on women in childbirth and finding it unsatisfactory in various ways, Simpson, with his two assistants, tried, one November evening, inhaling a similar but different chemical, chloroform. A listener in the next room noted how their talk grew 'louder and louder; a moment more and then all was quiet — and then *crash*. The inhaling party slipped off their chairs and flopped on the floor unconscious.'

James Simpson experiments with chloroform.

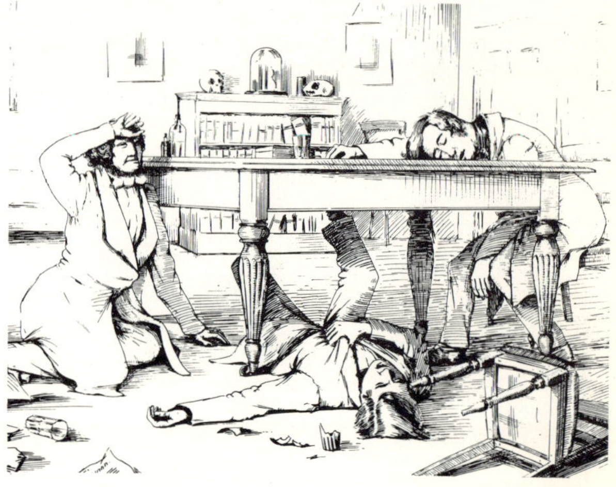

The first operation to be performed under an anaesthetic in the British Isles. The picture is a reconstruction and some people shown as present were not actually there. Before anaesthetics a surgeon usually needed at least two assistants to hold the patient down, so violent were the poor victim's struggles. One result of this was that professional surgeons tended to be huge, burly men, rather like wrestlers. Robert Liston, the surgeon in this picture, was famous throughout England for once having amputated a leg without any help whatsoever!

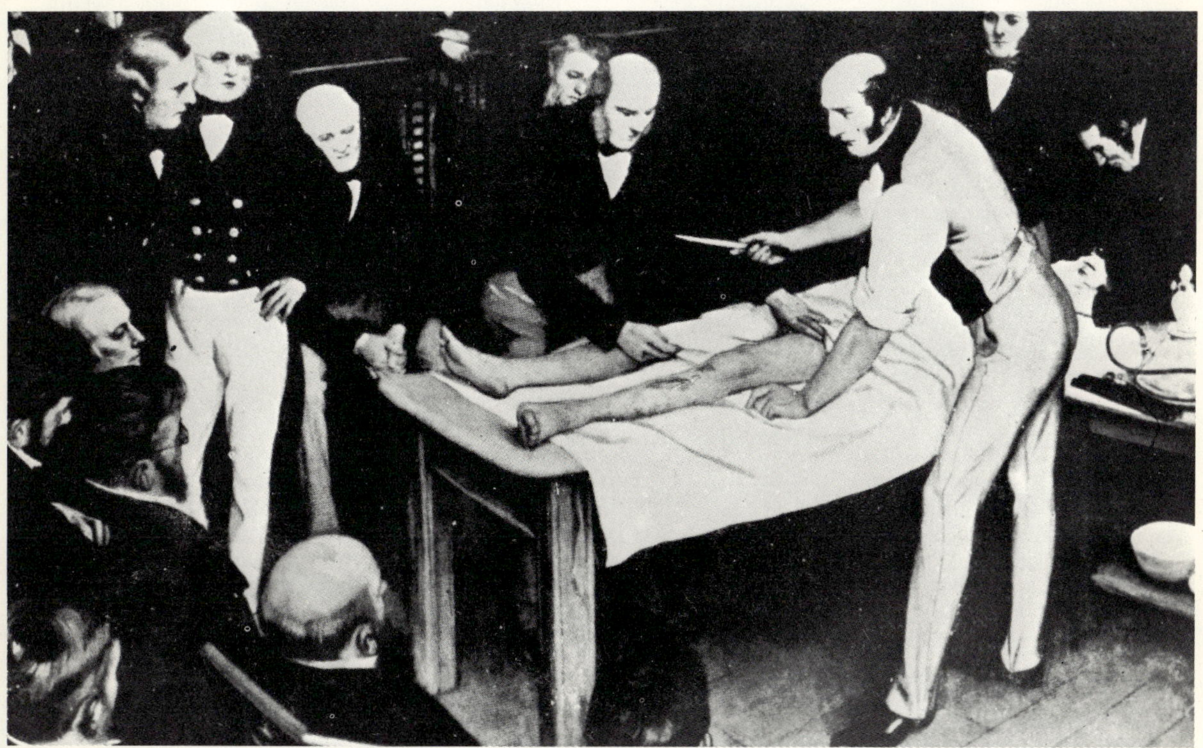

Within a fortnight Simpson had tried chloroform on fifty patients, with excellent results, but instead of being praised for the great blessing he had brought humanity, he was publicly attacked by the Scottish clergy for having discovered 'a decoy of Satan', which would 'rob God of the deep and earnest cries which arise in time of trouble for help'. Even the *Lancet* wrote in 1853 that 'in no case could it be justifiable to administer chloroform in a perfectly ordinary labour', but the argument was really settled by Queen Victoria, who accepted what she later called 'that blessed chloroform' during the birth of Prince Leopold in the same year. The anaesthetist was Dr John Snow, the first doctor in London to specialize in anaesthetics.

The most progressive doctors and the best hospitals gladly began to use anaesthetics without delay. The first painless operation at the Westminster Hospital took place in January 1847, on a woman suffering from abdominal growths. An eye-witness described how:

> The morbid growths were then dexterously shaved away . . . without any expression of pain on the part of the patient and without any signs of suffering apparent on her countenance. . . . On the completion of this operation, some wine and water was given to the patient, who seemed awakening from a dream. . . . After sundry ejaculations of wonder and surprise, she turned her head on her pillow and recognized one of the physicians as a 'real man' and discovered, to her infinite delight, that she was still a denizen of earth.

Anaesthesia

No one today need have a surgical operation without an anaesthetic. This has generally been true for the last hundred years, but even before the discovery of ether and chloroform, surgeons knew how to lessen pain — though not to eliminate it — by giving the patient narcotics, such as opium or Indian hemp, or alcohol or by applying ice and snow to the affected parts. None of these methods, however, were very effective, and often no attempt at all was made to anaesthetize the patient.

Today, with barbiturates to make the patient drowsy, nitrous oxide to produce complete unconsciousness and curare to relax the muscles, the surgeon's work is made much easier.

1799 Humphry Davy discovered that nitrous oxide (known as 'laughing gas') could make a patient unconscious. He suggested that it might be used in surgical operations, but the idea was not taken up.

1824 Henry Hill Hickman, a Shropshire doctor, amputated the limbs of animals previously made unconscious with carbon dioxide, but no one paid serious attention to his work.

1842 An American doctor, Crawford W. Long, removed a small tumour from a patient who had been anaesthetized with ether. His series of eight successful operations between 1843 and 1846 were not publicized until 1849.

1844 Horace Wells, a dentist in Connecticut, U.S.A., had one of his own teeth extracted painlessly after inhaling nitrous oxide. He committed suicide in 1848 after failing to impress the medical profession with his technique.

1846 (16 October) William Morton, a Boston dentist who had started his career as Wells' assistant, established anaesthesia on firm grounds when he and a surgeon successfully used ether during a major operation at the Massachusetts General Hospital. Morton had seen nitrous oxide not only as a useful aid in dentistry, but also as a way of relieving pain in major surgery. Finding that the safe limit of anaesthesia with nitrous oxide was only about a minute, he tried out the effects of liquid ether.
(21 December) Robert Liston, a surgeon at University College Hospital, London, performed the first major operation in Britain to be carried out under ether.

1847 Sir James Simpson experimented with chloroform on himself and two assistants, and went on to use it successfully on a number of patients. Public opinion was divided on the ethics of anaesthesia — some people objecting that it interfered with nature.

1853 John Snow, a London doctor, used chloroform with Queen Victoria's permission at the birth of her son, Prince Leopold. Opposition from the public and some quarters of the medical profession gradually decreased after this.
The hypodermic syringe invented. It was first used for injecting morphine to produce anaesthesia in 1855.

1874 Middlesex Hospital appointed its first anaesthetist.

1884 Cocaine first used as a local anaesthetic (that is, part of the body is numbed whilst keeping the patient conscious). Sigmund Freud, the founder of psychoanalysis, discovered this use of cocaine, but until he prescribed it for a friend who became a confirmed addict, he had no idea of its side-effects. Today, it is only used in certain types of eye and throat surgery.

1892 A gas and oxygen apparatus invented. It had been found that nitrous oxide on its own made a patient unconscious, but did not bring about the necessary muscular relaxation, nor did it entirely avoid the danger of asphyxia. It was therefore mixed with oxygen.

1905 Novacocaine, an improvement on cocaine, first used in Germany.

1942 Curare, a South American poison which temporarily paralyses the muscles, first used in addition to an anaesthetic. Sir Walter Raleigh, in 1596, was one of the first Europeans to describe the 'poysoned herbes' from one of which curare is obtained. A century and a half later a Frenchman, La Condamine, described how he had seen it used by an Indian tribe to tip their arrows and blow-pipe darts on hunting expeditions. Experiments were then made by La Condamine and other scientists to see how it worked. It was found that a curarized victim's heart continues beating for up to two hours after unconsciousness.

Yet seven years later in 1854 the Chief of Medical Staff of the British Army in the Crimea was still declaring that 'the smart use of the knife is a powerful stimulant and it is much better to hear a man bawl lustily than to see him sink silently into the grave', and there were many old fashioned civilian surgeons who spoke approvingly of 'a good healthy scream'.

Death in the wards

Anaesthetics made it possible to carry out more and more difficult operations, and so the number of hospital deaths after they came into use actually increased. A common cause of death was blood-poisoning, which showed itself in fever, and might lead to pains in the joints and, sometimes, a rash, perhaps with multiple abscesses developing in distant parts of the body, like the lungs, liver and brain. Some patients succumbed to tetanus, or lockjaw, during which the body was racked with spasms and the jaw and face became locked in a ghastly forced smile, until the patient, who was still conscious, died from heart failure or was suffocated by the paralysis of his breathing muscles. One skin infection, erysipelas, marked by a red rash and increased temperature, was notorious for spreading with astonishing speed through a whole ward or hospital, but most dreaded of all, and equally infectious, was hospital gangrene, which killed the tissues round the wound, which became purplish-black, and then spread over the whole body. The surgeon who smelt the pus suppurating in the wound or saw the ominous purplish-black skin around it knew at once that he was likely to lose in the ward yet another patient whose life he had saved in the operating theatre. As yet, however, he did not know why. And just as doctors who could not understand how cholera spread in the slums blamed 'the poisonous miasma' in the air, so in the wards 'hospital miasma' was held responsible for epidemics of gangrene.

By now many doctors in many countries were beginning to doubt this simple explanation. One of the first was Ignaz Semmelweiss, who lived from 1818 to 1865, and who noticed in Vienna in 1846 that one obstetric ward in the hospital where he worked had such a high death rate from puerperal fever, which attacked women after childbirth, that they begged with tears in their eyes not to be placed there. This ward was, Semmelweiss realized, the one which medical students visited directly after working in the dissecting room, and without washing their hands. The death rate in another ward, looked after by midwives, who did wash their hands before every delivery, was far lower. Then one day one of Semmelweiss's professors himself died after cutting himself during a dissection. His 'fatal symptoms,' wrote the young doctor, 'unveiled to my mind an identity with those I had so often noticed in the death-bed of puerperal cases.' He put up a notice on the entrance to the clinic:

> From today, 15 May 1847, any doctor or student coming from the post mortem room must, before entering the maternity wards, wash his hands thoroughly in the basin of chlorinated water placed at the entrance. This order applies to everyone, without exception.

Although some of his professors supported Semmelweiss most doctors were furious at his 'interference', even though within a few months the death rate among the mothers had dropped by three-quarters and within two years by nine-tenths. Semmelweiss went home to Budapest, where he cut the death rate from puerperal fever in the local maternity hospital to under one patient in a hundred. Here, too, there was bitter opposition to his reforms. He could not even get clean sheets provided for each patient until he had dumped a heap of dirty, evil-smelling sheets, which had been used by one patient after another, on the desk of the hospital's director. In 1861 Semmelweiss virtually

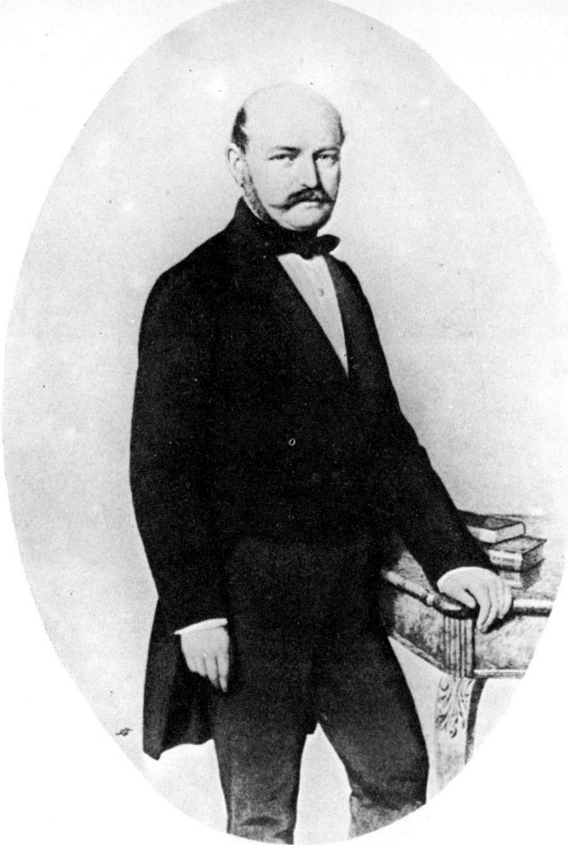

Ignaz Philipp Semmelweiss, the Hungarian doctor who pioneered antiseptic methods in hospitals.

Oliver Wendell Holmes, an American doctor and man of letters, who was one of the pioneers of anaesthesia. It was Holmes who coined the word 'anaesthesia'.

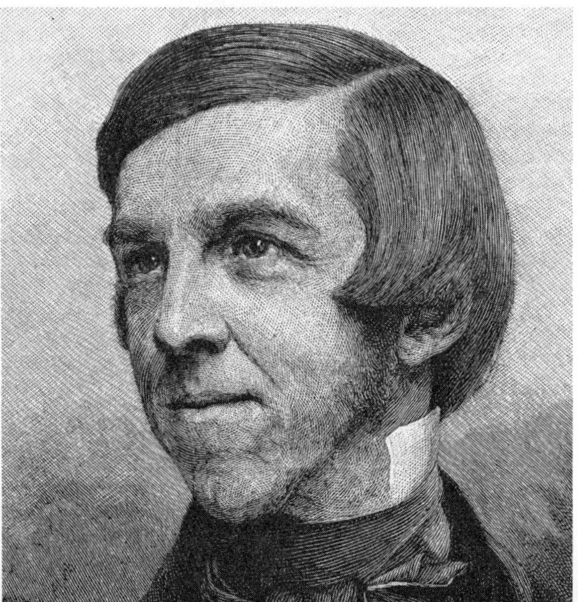

declared war on his obstinate colleagues, in a famous open letter to a leading doctor in Vienna who refused to practise his methods. Semmelweiss accused him of sharing in the responsibility for 'thousands upon thousands of deaths', urged him 'to halt this slaughter' and threatened that if he took no action 'I shall denounce you before God and the world as a murderer'. But even this produced no results and four years later Semmelweiss died insane, ironically enough of blood-poisoning, the very disease he had helped to conquer. Today one of the great Viennese hospitals bears his name.

At about the same time that Semmelweiss was fighting his uphill battle against prejudice in Europe another doctor, Oliver Wendell Holmes (1809–94) was encountering similar hostility in America. In 1843 he published *The Contagiousness of Puerperal Fever*, as the opening shot in his campaign for 'clean hands' in midwifery, but his work was discredited after a doctor had apparently carried the disease to four of his patients, despite washing his hands. (The explanation, not realized at the time, was that soap and water alone were not always enough to kill an infection.)

The germ-theory of disease

The discovery which finally carried medicine a giant stride forward was made not by a doctor but by a chemist, Louis Pasteur. Pasteur was born in 1822, the son of a tanner, and after working as a schoolmaster he became Professor of Chemistry at Lille University, where he was asked to study the reasons why wine went sour. After brilliant research, Pasteur established in 1864 that the cause was not 'spontaneous', that it did not just arise of itself, but from a tiny micro-organism, far too small to be seen, which was transmitted through the air. In later work on other diseases, affecting silkworms, sheep and dogs, Pasteur proved conclusively that diseases never did

A brilliantly simple experiment devised by Pasteur to show that organisms are carried in the air and that they must be heavier than air. The flask on the left contains sterilized water, and it remains sterilized because the organisms cannot travel uphill through the tube. Break off the tube and the water becomes infected within two days. Pasteur also showed that the number of organisms was not the same everywhere: there were more in the air of a busy street than on the top of a mountain.

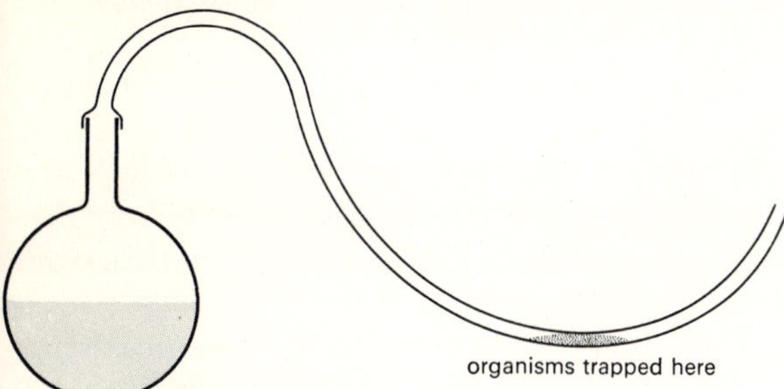

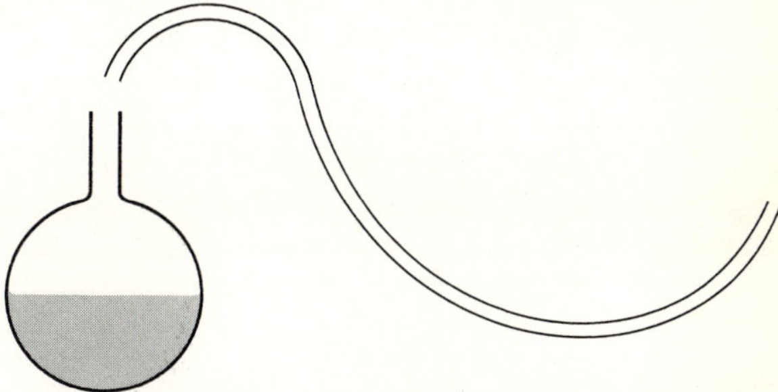

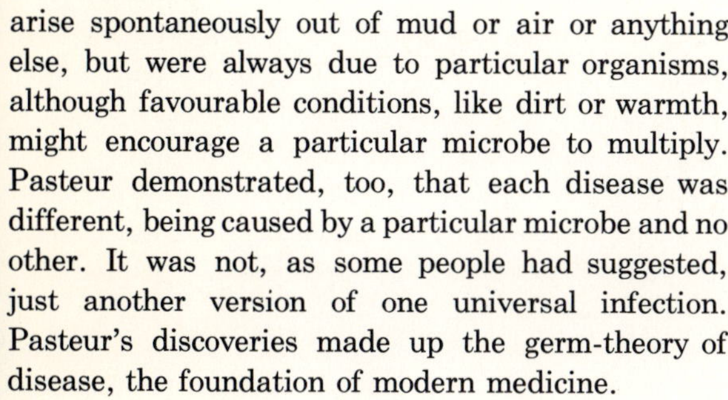

arise spontaneously out of mud or air or anything else, but were always due to particular organisms, although favourable conditions, like dirt or warmth, might encourage a particular microbe to multiply. Pasteur demonstrated, too, that each disease was different, being caused by a particular microbe and no other. It was not, as some people had suggested, just another version of one universal infection. Pasteur's discoveries made up the germ-theory of disease, the foundation of modern medicine.

Surgery made safe

While Pasteur had been perfecting his theory in France, a young surgeon called Joseph Lister had been puzzling over the problem of hospital infection in Glasgow. Lister had been born in Essex in 1827, the son of a comfortably-off wine-merchant who, as a hobby, studied the use of the microscope. Lister had thus many advantages denied to Pasteur and by seventeen he was a medical student at University College Hospital in London, where he watched the famous 'anaesthetic' operation by Robert Liston already described. By the time he was thirty-three, Lister had risen to be Professor of Surgery at Glasgow, where he was soon greatly respected. His students idolized him, calling him 'The Chief'; his patients, to whom he was always sympathetic and considerate, admired and trusted him. But still, despite all his care and the skilful operations he performed on them, many of them contracted gangrene and died.

Lister once wrote of himself, 'As to brilliant talent, I know I do not possess it; but I must try to make up as far as I can by perseverance.' In 1865 he read of Pasteur's researches and suddenly it dawned upon him that it was not the air itself, as doctors had so long believed, which spread hospital gangrene, it was the germs in the air. Pasteur had shown that harmful micro-organisms could be destroyed by heat, by filtration and by antiseptics, and Lister realized that it was the third of these which offered the most practical way of protecting a surgical wound from infection. He decided to use for the purpose a strong disinfectant, carbolic acid, which was known to be effective against sewage, and in 1865 made his first experiment, on a boy of eleven, with a bandage soaked in carbolic acid. The patient was suffering from a compound fracture of the thigh, in which broken bones had pierced the skin. This was just the type of case which most often ended in gangrene.

Although this first experiment was only a partial success (the acid burned the patient's skin) by the following year Lister had developed a better method and tried it on another compound fracture, of the leg. 'It is now eight days since the accident', he was soon able to write to his father, 'and the patient has been going on exactly as if the fracture were a simple one,' i.e. one which had not broken the skin. A year later he had even better news: 'Fifteen cases of compound fracture were treated by my house surgeon . . . and every one of these men and women are living with their limbs on.'

In this year, 1867, Lister published his researches to the world in the *Lancet*. Curiously enough, their importance was realized abroad long before most British doctors had accepted them. This was partly due to Lister's muddled style, but also because many doctors who copied his methods badly found the death rate as high as before. Soon, like John Snow, Lister was actually being criticized for holding up medical progress. Dr James Simpson, who had first used chloroform, was one of his harshest critics and a poll conducted by the *Lancet* in 1869 showed that the leading London surgeons regarded Lister's precautions against infection as 'quite useless' or 'meddlesome'.

On the continent, however, it was a different story. One influential German professor of surgery had become so desperate at the various forms of infection raging through his hospital that 'for a full quarter of a year no one dared to touch a knife in the surgical clinic', and he had even suggested pulling the whole building down. The change, once he tried Lister's methods, was astonishing; seventy-five patients suffering from compound fractures all recovered, and out of 139 he lost only four. Meanwhile at Munich another doctor had become equally desperate. 'Hospital gangrene, gnawing at the wound like a wild beast' had attacked 50 per cent of his surgical cases in 1872 and 80 per cent in 1874. He sent his assistant to Edinburgh to study Lister's methods. By the following year, so remarkable was the change that he was writing of 'Lister's great discovery', which was, he said, 'being greeted by the whole civilized world as an enormous advance'.

In 1877 Lister moved to King's College, London. Opinion in the capital was still divided about the value of his methods. Guy's Hospital had been using them in every ward since 1873, but at the Westminster Hospital only one surgeon believed in them. Elsewhere diehard doctors could still get a laugh from their students by slamming the door of the operating theatre 'to keep Mr Lister's germs out'. At a great International Medical Congress in London in 1881 a doctor from St Bartholomew's Hospital publicly ridiculed the whole antiseptic system, in front of Pasteur, Lister and Robert Koch, whose work will be mentioned shortly. It was left to a German surgeon to remind the British doctors that 'England may be proud that it was one of her sons whose name is indissolubly bound up with the greatest advance that surgery has ever made.'

The Lister spray

One reason why many surgeons were unwilling to take antiseptic precautions was the Lister spray, a machine operated at first by hand and then by a small engine, which pumped out carbolic acid to kill the infection in the air. Working near the spray was unpleasant and, if you breathed in the vapour, it could be actually harmful. By 1890 Lister himself had realized it was in any case almost useless. (Its disappearance robbed the medical students of the time-honoured joke of calling out 'Let us spray!' as the machine started up.) By now Lister and his colleagues had discovered, too, that it was not air which transmitted germs from patient to patient so much as the medical staff themselves. Often up to now doctors and students had gone from patient to patient without washing their hands using the same instruments and the same piece of sponge. Now, under the impetus of Lister's campaign, much greater care was taken in hospitals everywhere.

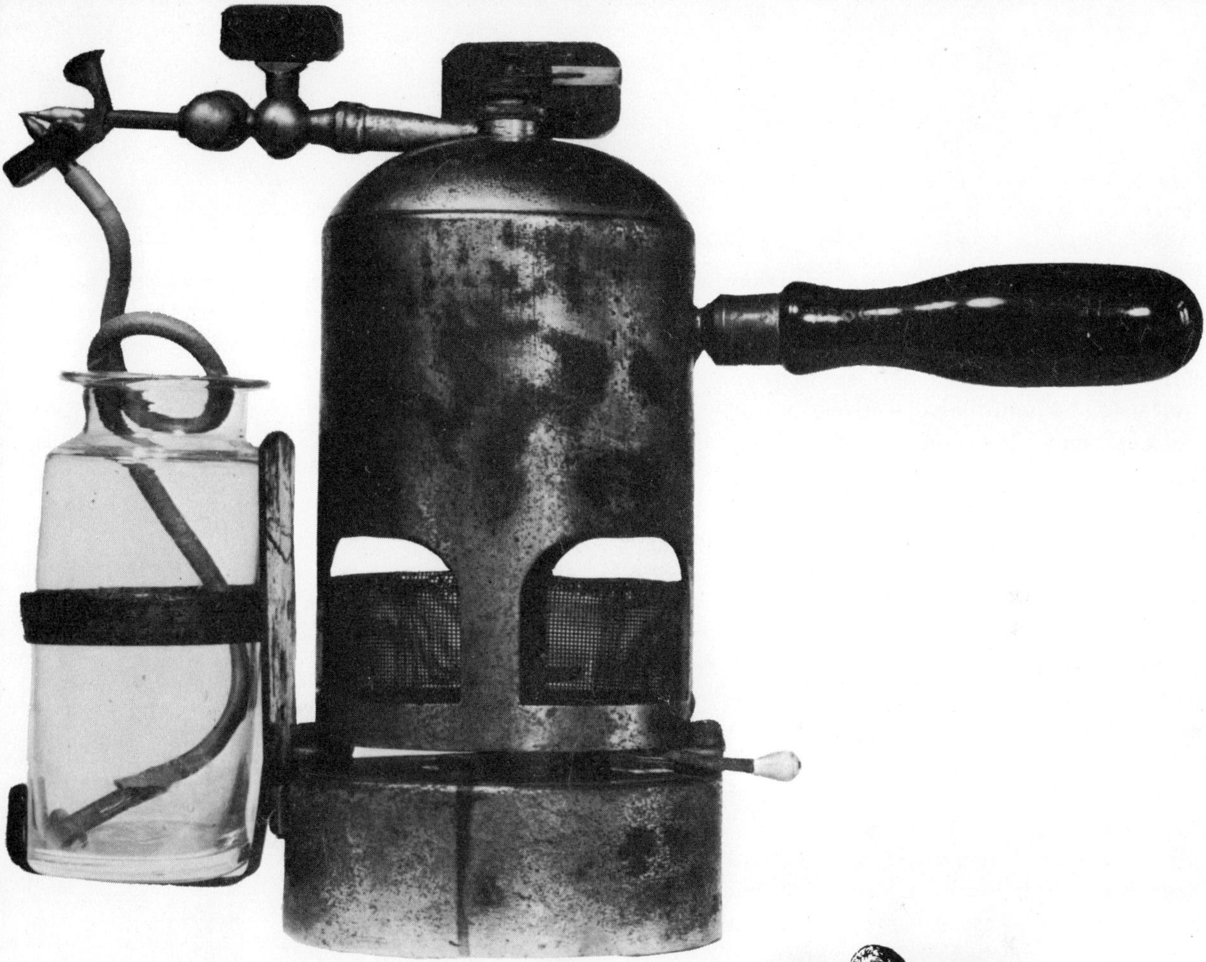

Above The Lister carbolic spray.

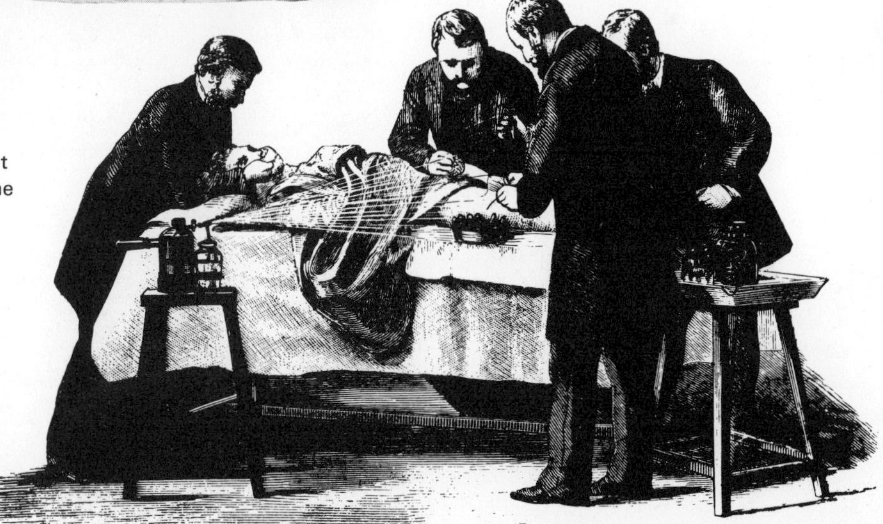

Right The spray in use. It was not a very efficient way of keeping the patient free from infection, and it can hardly have been pleasant for the surgeon to work under a shower.

The greatest change of all occurred in the operating theatre. Today we are so accustomed to the picture of the spotlessly clean stainless steel operating table, surrounded by doctors and nurses in white gowns, caps and face masks, with the surgeon wearing rubber gloves and boots and using carefully sterilized instruments, that it is hard to realize how different the operating theatre looked a century ago. At that time the operating table was made of wood and the surgeon operated in his ordinary clothes, probably wearing an old frock coat to protect them, with the ligatures he used for stitching up the wound tucked into his buttonhole. Some surgeons were proud of wearing a coat so thick with blood and dirt that it would stand up by itself, and the same old blanket was used to cover patient after patient and seldom washed.

Between 1867 and 1900 all this changed, assisted by the development in Germany around 1887 of a machine for sterilizing dressings and instruments by heat or steam. It became realized that the ideal was not so much antisepsis, defeating infection, as asepsis, ensuring that infection was never present. As late as 1900, however, a nurse at the London Hospital saw, she later recalled, surgeons working without gloves and with sweat dripping from their beards into the open incision, while at another hospital a surgeon, when asked to wear rubber boots while operating, jovially asked if he were expected to stand inside the patient.

Except among an obstinate few, Lister's ideas had everywhere triumphed long before his death in 1912 at the age of eighty-four. By now his great achievements had been fully appreciated. In 1897 he was created a peer by Queen Victoria, and a few years later her son, Edward VII, who had recently been operated on for appendicitis, told him, 'Lord Lister, I know that if it had not been for you and your work I would not have been here today.' Lister perhaps valued even more the tribute of a French doctor who told him 'you have driven back death itself'. By the time of Lister's death more than ten times as many operations were being performed as in 1867 and surgeons, for the first time, were able to operate without fear on every part of the human body.

Lord Lister. A portrait in very official style, as President of the Royal Society.

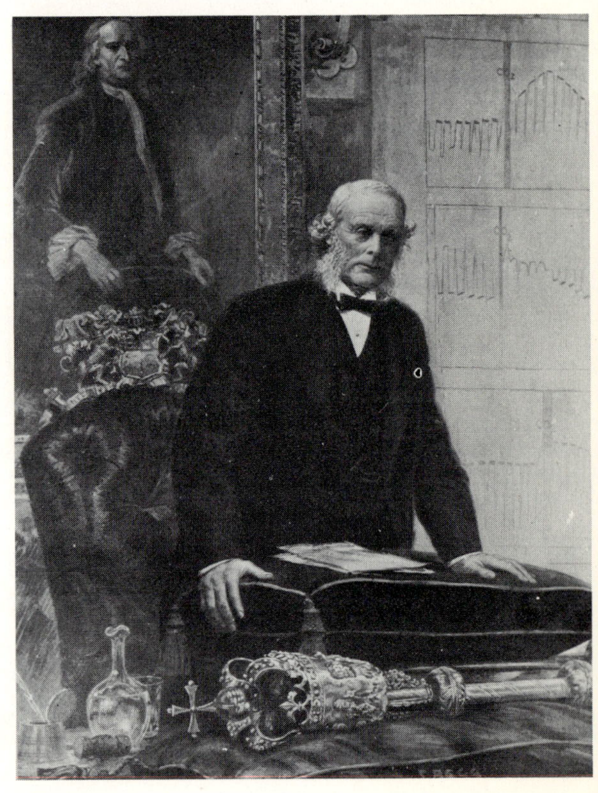

The progress of surgery

1804 Grafts of small areas of skin first carried out.

1825 Chlorine solution first used for purposes of disinfection.

1865 Joseph Lister, having read of Pasteur's discoveries, pioneered the use of antiseptics in surgery.

1871 George Lawson, an English surgeon, was the first to transplant large areas of skin.

1880 First successful series of operations for appendicitis. The first appendectomy was done as early as 1736, but the risk of infection and wrong diagnosis had prevented further progress.

1885 Experimental heart-lung machine invented in Germany.

1886 First operation performed under sterile, or aseptic, conditions — an improvement on antisepsis.

1887 A machine for sterilizing dressings and instruments by heat or steam developed in Germany.

1894 Surgeons began to use rubber gloves for operations.

1895 Röntgen discovered X-rays. This enabled surgeons to look into a patient's body without opening it up, thus making diagnosis much easier.

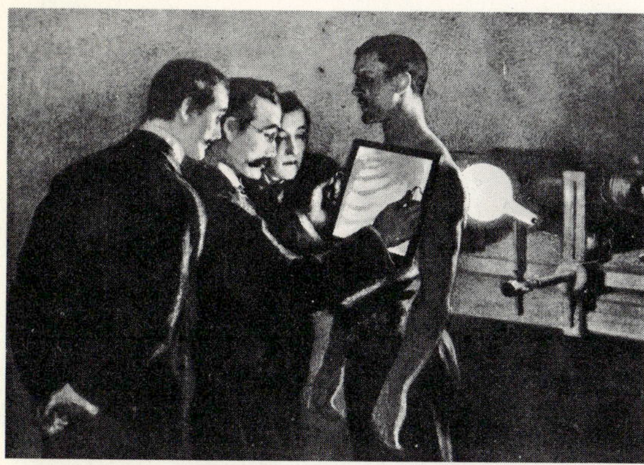

The first radiologists, unaware of the effects of lengthy exposure to X-rays, suffered painful and slow-healing skin burns. Some, in fact, died of skin cancer and leukaemia.

1896 An open heart wound successfully stitched up in Germany.

1898 Pierre and Marie Curie discovered radium. Radiotherapy was later used in the treatment of cancer: radioactive needles are implanted near the cancer site and give off intense radiation which kills the cancer cells. X-rays are also used for this purpose.

1899 Gauze face-masks first used in the operating theatre.

1900 Karl Landsteiner discovered the division of blood into groups. This discovery greatly improved the technique of blood transfusion.

1903 Willem Einthoven developed the electrocardiograph. This gives a graphic tracing of the electric currents produced by the contraction of the heart muscles.

1907 Alexis Carrel devised a way of connecting together blood vessels in animals. This technique enabled him to transplant organs and limbs, though only in animals.

1915 The 'Carrel-Dakin solution' made it possible to treat infection in deep-seated war wounds. Bone grafts first used as internal splints.

1929 A German doctor invented the cardiac catheter for examining the heart by means of a tube passed along a vein.

1938 National Blood Transfusion Service founded.

1944 First successful kidney machine developed.

1950 First kidney transplant successfully performed in Chicago.

1953 First successful operation using a heart-lung machine.

1968 First heart transplant successfully carried out in South Africa by a team of surgeons led by Professor Christian Barnard, though the patient died eighteen months later.

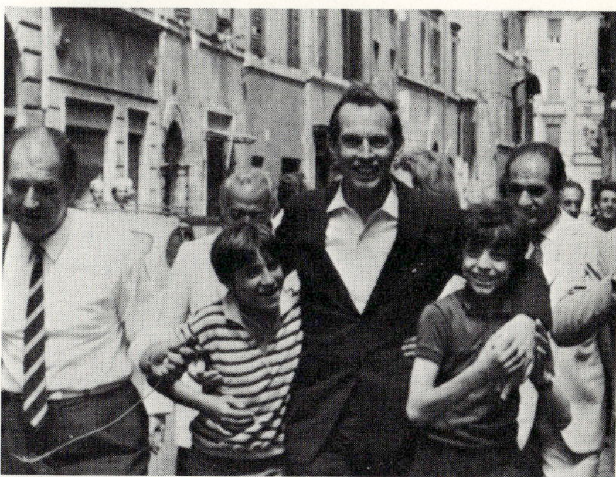

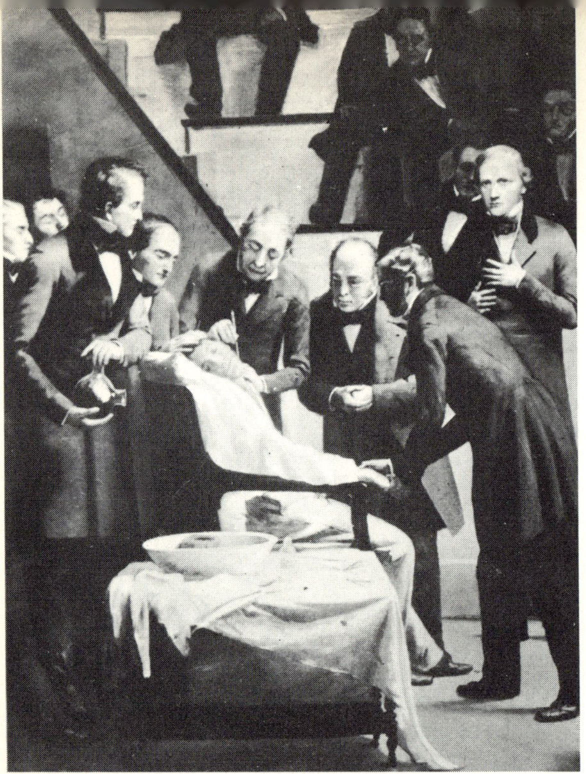

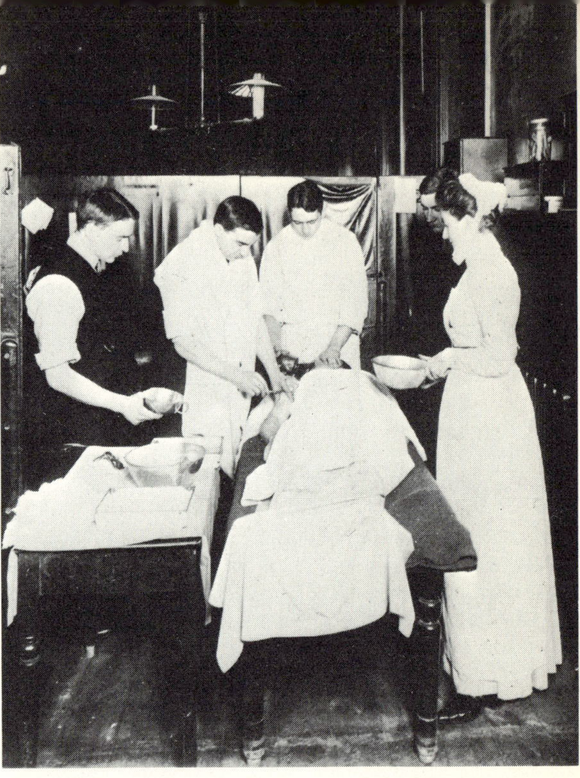

Three operating theatres. Left above is an American operating theatre in 1846: it shows the first operation anywhere using ether. Drs Morton and Warren remove a tumour on the jaw of one Gilbert Abbott. Above is the theatre at St Bartholomew's Hospital, around 1910, and below is a modern operating theatre.

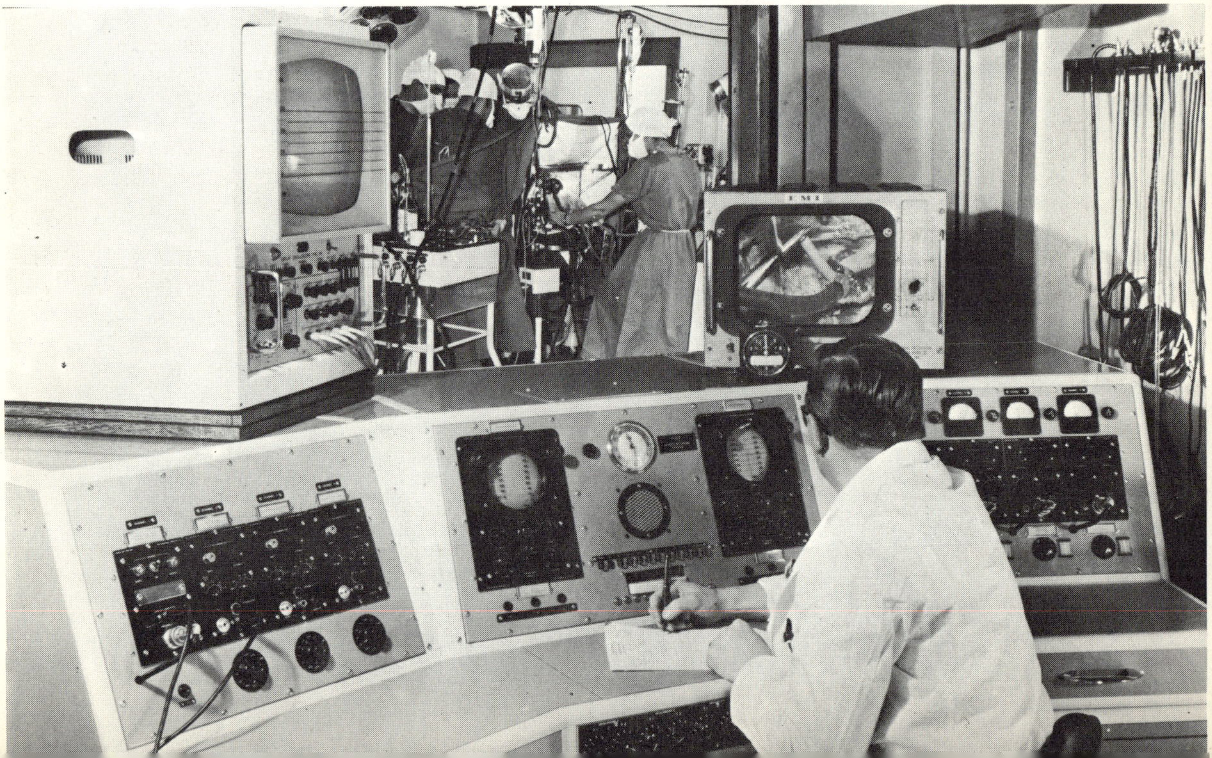

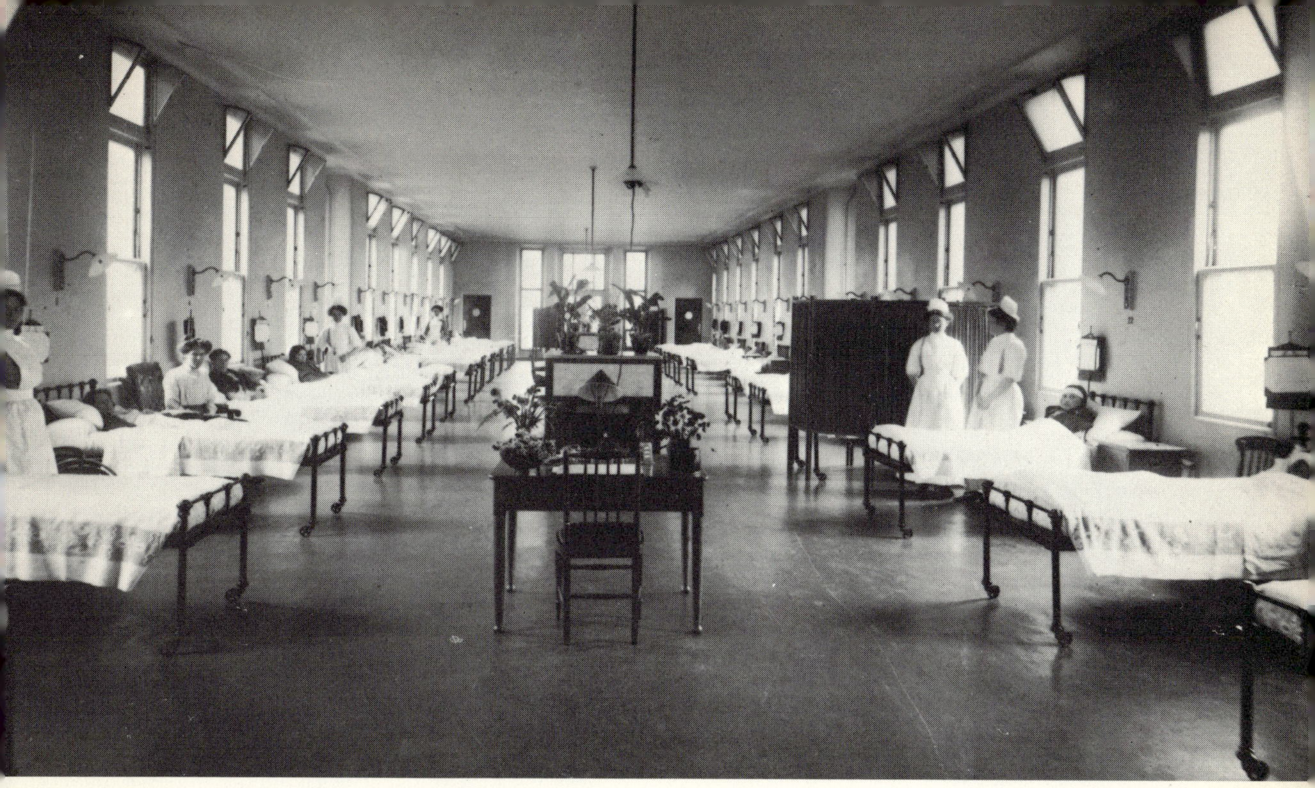

King's College Hospital in 1914, and below Hillingdon Hospital, Middlesex today.

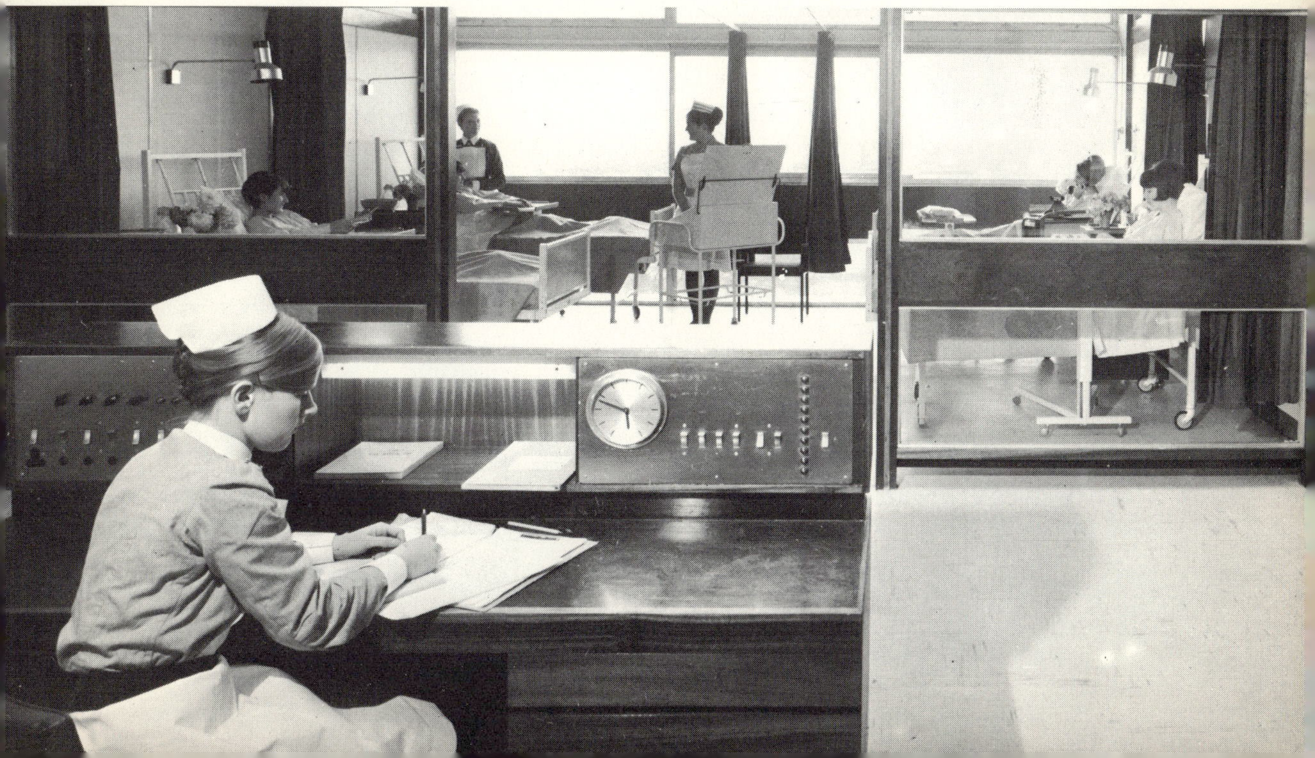

6 Immunization and drugs

Robert Koch

Pasteur had proved that microbes existed, Lister had shown how harmful ones could be destroyed, but no one had so far discovered how to identify the different types of germ. Today when a diagnosis is in doubt a specimen from the patient is automatically sent to the laboratory to be positively identified, but in the 1870s a doctor had to wait for the symptoms to develop and even then he might guess wrong. To name and classify the chief varieties of microbe was essential for further medical progress and this was the contribution of Robert Koch. Koch was born in Clausthal, Germany, in 1843, one of thirteen children of a mining engineer, and, after serving as an army surgeon during the Franco-Prussian war, became a general practitioner in a country district in 1872. Already he was passionately interested in medical research, but there was no money to spare for expensive equipment, so his wife curtained off part of his surgery as a makeshift laboratory, and saved coins in a beer mug to buy him a good microscope, while his daughter made pets out of the guinea pigs, mice and monkeys he kept in the garden for his experiments. Koch's great chance came when, after being appealed to by the local farmers to help them fight an epidemic of anthrax, which caused their sheep to turn black and die, he succeeded in identifying the bacillus responsible and showed how the disease could be halted. The German government, recognizing his outstanding abilities, installed him in a fine laboratory in Berlin and here he developed methods of cultivating and classifying bacteria which are still in use. He also isolated many bacilli for the first time, including, in 1884, the 'comma bacillus', so called from its shape, which spread cholera, a disease in which he had been interested since as a young man of twenty-three he had helped to fight a serious epidemic in Hamburg. He rounded off John Snow's great discovery, and further strengthened the germ-theory of disease, by proving that 'Cholera does not come into being spontaneously. . . . It is a disease that attacks only those who have swallowed the comma bacillus.' He finally showed that tales of a 'poisonous miasma' or of a common cause of epidemics were nonsense, demonstrating that 'each particular disease is caused by one microbe and one alone'.

Curiously enough, as had happened to John Snow, some leading doctors refused to accept his theory. One obstinate old miasmatist actually asked Koch for a flask containing comma bacilli and drank the contents to prove they were not to blame — and, almost miraculously, escaped. By now, however, the evidence implicating the comma bacillus and the water supply was overwhelming. The last great epidemic in Western Europe, in Hamburg in 1892, really settled the matter, for Koch showed that almost all the 8,200 deaths occurred in the part of the city served by a contaminated water supply, just as in Soho in 1854 and East London in 1866. This was almost the end of the miasmatic theory, which had done so much to obstruct medical progress throughout the nineteenth century.

Having solved the mystery of cholera, Koch went on to greater triumphs, travelling all over the world to study the diseases of both men and cattle and everywhere making discoveries which brought a sharp fall in the death rate. Unlike John Snow and Joseph Lister, he was a far from likeable man, being arrogant and short-tempered. But, whatever his character, Koch's place in medical history is secure. By the time he died, of heart disease in 1910, the science of bacteriology was firmly established, and largely because of his efforts.

Men against microbes

When Koch began his work there was still much misunderstanding of the nature of disease, though he had

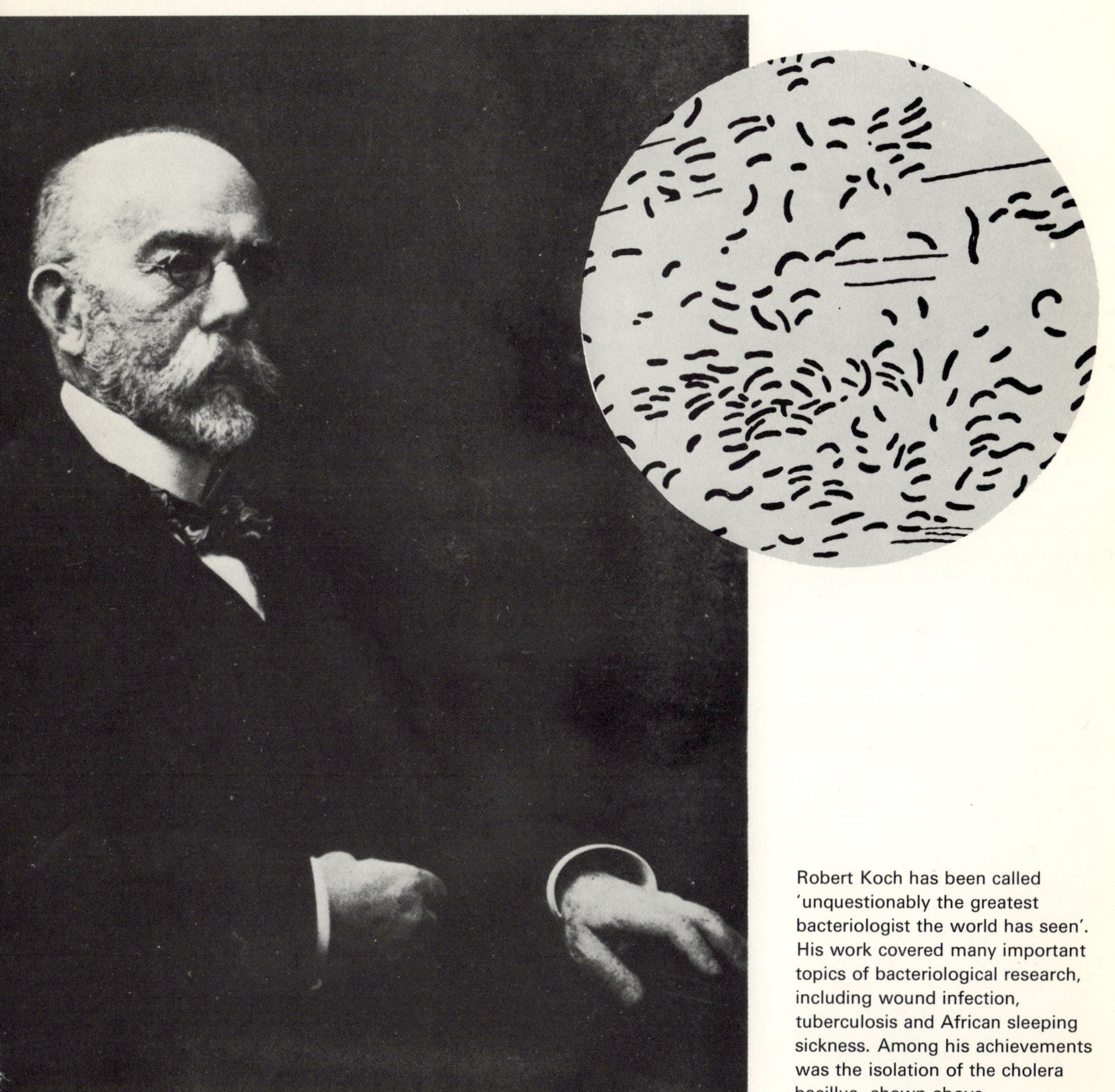

Robert Koch has been called 'unquestionably the greatest bacteriologist the world has seen'. His work covered many important topics of bacteriological research, including wound infection, tuberculosis and African sleeping sickness. Among his achievements was the isolation of the cholera bacillus, shown above.

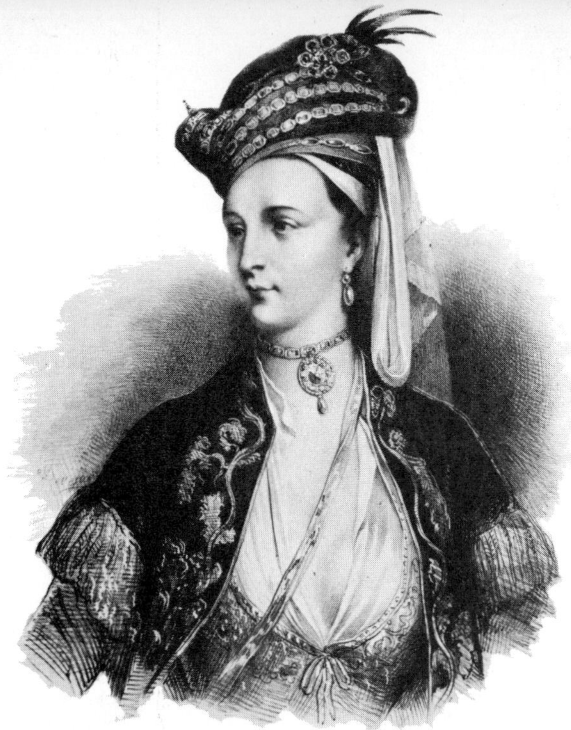

It was well known that once someone had had smallpox they could not have the disease again. Physicians in Turkey had been experimenting with methods of immunizing people by exposing them to infection from people who had only a mild attack of the disease. It was Lady Mary Wortley Montagu (above) who brought this method to people's attention in Europe in 1718. But the Turkish way of doing it was dangerous, and many people died from this method of inoculation. It was Edward Jenner (below) who discovered that someone who had had cowpox (a much milder disease) was just as well protected as someone who had had smallpox itself.

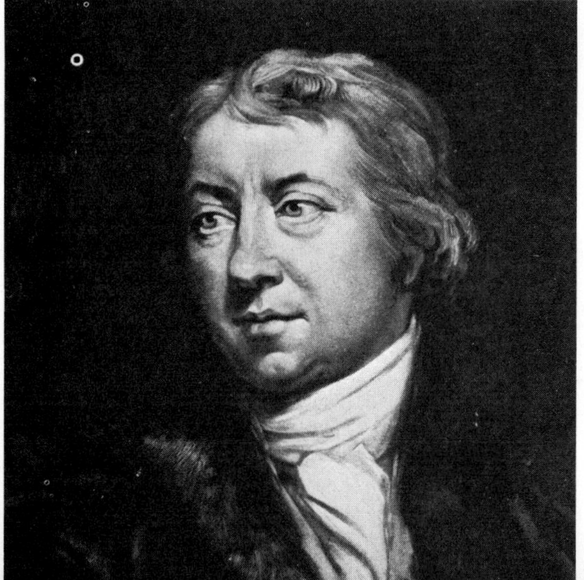

finally destroyed the belief that epidemics had a common origin. By the time of his death a great deal was known about the identity of many bacteria and their behaviour and everywhere efforts were being made to make them allies as well as enemies of man. The idea of immunizing human beings against a disease by giving them a mild form of it was nothing new. As long ago as 1796 Dr Edward Jenner had begun vaccinating people against smallpox by deliberately infecting them with the related disease of cowpox, although he could not explain why this worked. Pasteur, who could, declared that 'We must immunize against the infectious diseases of which we can cultivate the causative micro-organisms' — hence the importance of bacteriologists like Koch who made it possible to produce in the laboratory the microbes required. After successfully immunizing hens and pigs against various diseases, Pasteur in 1881 successfully and publicly immunized against anthrax, the disease which had first made Koch's name, a flock of twenty-four sheep and six cows which, along with twenty-nine animals which had not been vaccinated, were deliberately infected with the disease. A few days later, as he approached the cattle pens, he was greeted with loud cheering from the crowd; all the vaccinated sheep and cows were well, the unvaccinated were almost all dead or dying. Pasteur now turned to the study of rabies, a rare but terrible disease, spread by mad dogs, which weeks, or even months, after the bite had healed, caused the victim to be seized by terrible convulsions as he struggled to swallow or breathe, until he died an agonizing death. Even today the organism which causes the disease is unknown and once it is established in the body there is no known cure. In 1890 Pasteur tried out his new vaccine on a young boy bitten by a mad dog, who Pasteur knew was bound to die if it failed. But the boy lived and years later became gate-keeper at the great Pasteur research institute in Paris named after the man who had saved him.

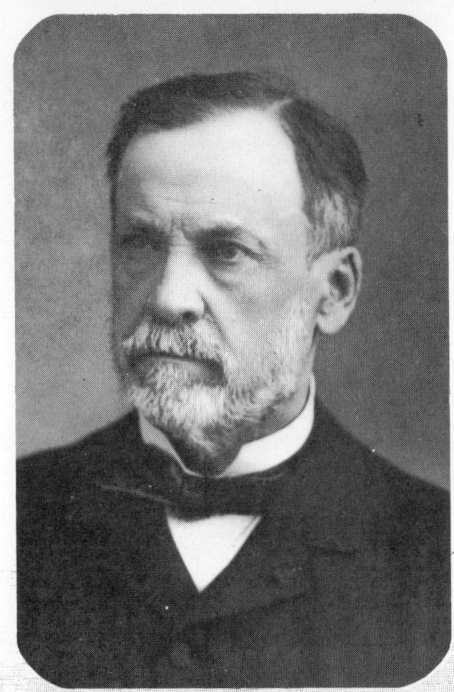

Louis Pasteur.

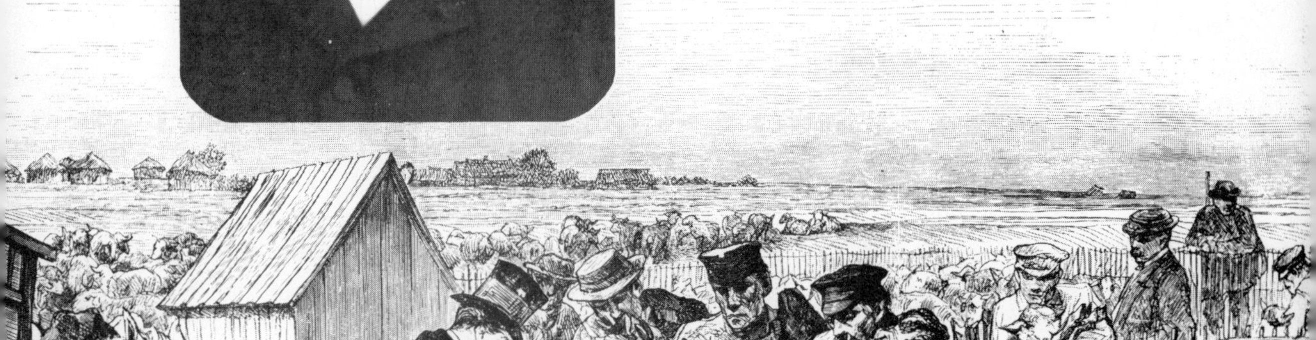

Anthrax is a very contagious disease which mostly affects animals, but occasionally people as well. In this engraving Pasteur demonstrates publicly the value of vaccination.

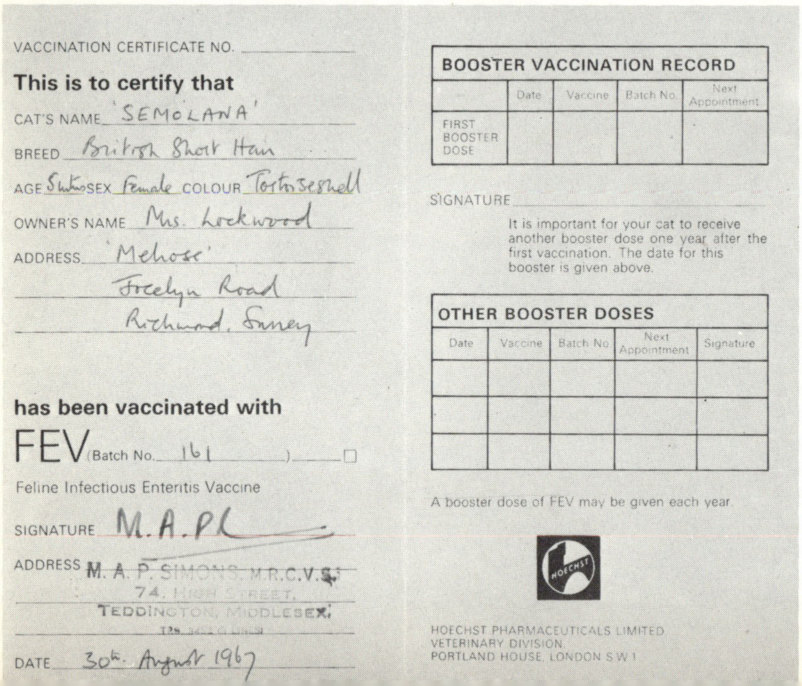

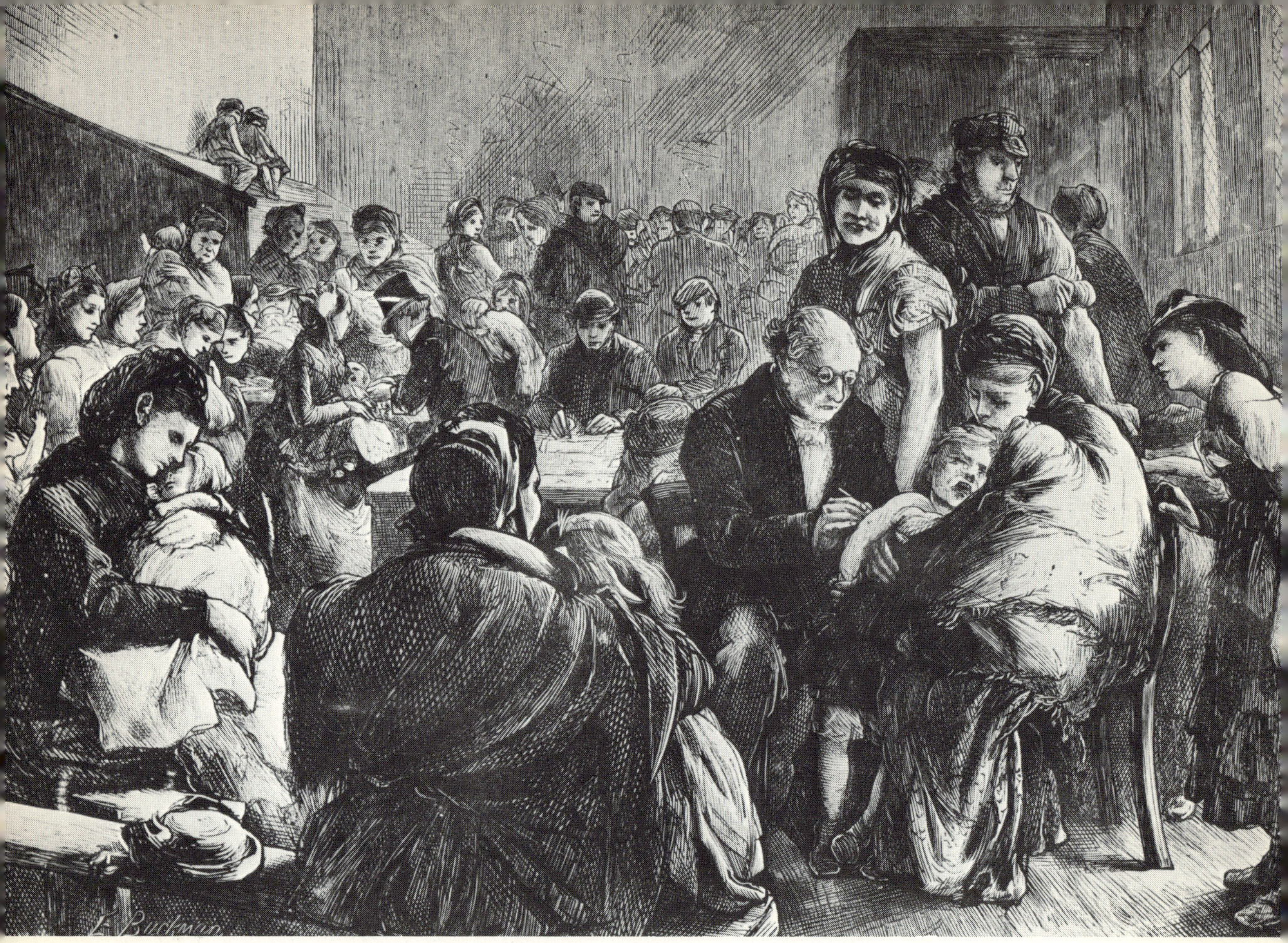

VACCINATION CERTIFICATE NO. ____________

This is to certify that

CAT'S NAME 'SEMOLANA'

BREED British Short Hair

AGE [illegible] SEX Female COLOUR Tortoiseshell

OWNER'S NAME Mrs. Lockwood

ADDRESS 'Melrose'
Jocelyn Road
Richmond, Surrey

has been vaccinated with

FEV (Batch No. 161) ______ ☐

Feline Infectious Enteritis Vaccine

SIGNATURE M. A. P[illegible]

ADDRESS M. A. P. SIMONS, M.R.C.V.S.
74, HIGH STREET,
TEDDINGTON, MIDDLESEX.

DATE 30th. August 1967

BOOSTER VACCINATION RECORD

	Date	Vaccine	Batch No.	Next Appointment
FIRST BOOSTER DOSE				

SIGNATURE ____________

It is important for your cat to receive another booster dose one year after the first vaccination. The date for this booster is given above.

OTHER BOOSTER DOSES

Date	Vaccine	Batch No.	Next Appointment	Signature

A booster dose of FEV may be given each year.

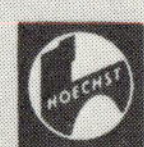

HOECHST PHARMACEUTICALS LIMITED
VETERINARY DIVISION
PORTLAND HOUSE, LONDON S.W.1

A District Vaccinator in the East End of London in 1871.

Left The benefits of vaccination are nowadays available to other creatures as well. This cat has been vaccinated against enteritis, an unpleasant and contagious disease which particularly affects cats.

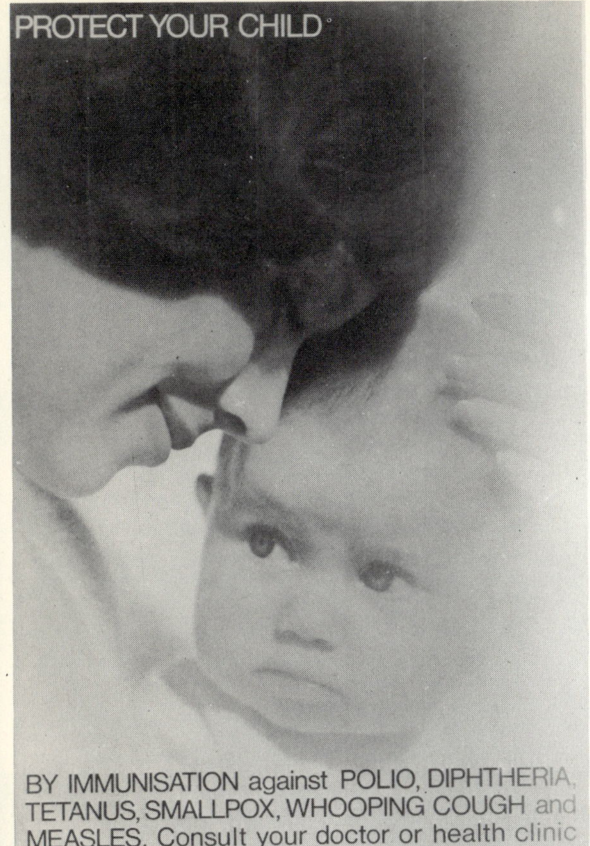

A modern poster persuading parents to ensure that they have their children vaccinated.

Deaths from diphtheria in England between 1938 and 1951 declined dramatically through immunization of children.

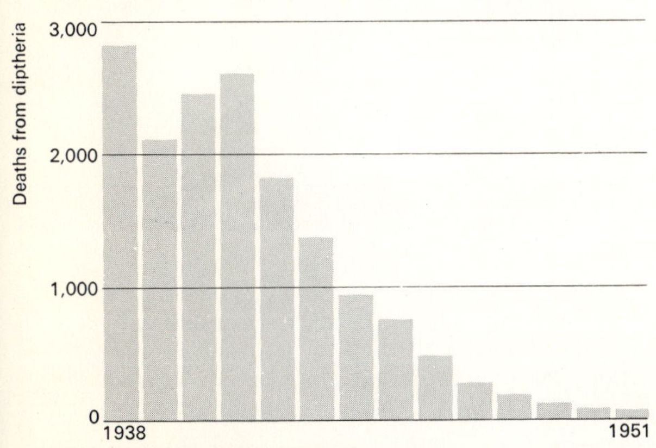

Immunization

Inoculation can be given before or after the onset of disease. To protect people from the commoner, quicker-acting diseases, the aim has always been to provide defence beforehand. In the last twenty years of the nineteenth century it was realized that immunization worked because an invading microbe caused the body to struggle to defend itself by producing anti-bodies to destroy the invader. If it was too weak to succeed, the disease triumphed. But if advance immunization was given in good time, the defending anti-bodies were produced in such numbers that the invading disease never had a chance to establish itself. In other words, the person concerned never 'caught' the disease at all. What had actually happened, of course, was that he *had* caught the disease but the waiting anti-bodies had prevented it doing him any harm.

As every type of bacteria is different, it took years of research to discover the best method to protect the body in each case. Much work was done both on 'active' immunization, which provides long-term protection, perhaps for a life-time, by stimulating the body to produce its own anti-bodies, and on 'passive' immunization, which provides the anti-bodies themselves, in a form known as 'anti-sera', for immediate assistance when infection has actually occurred. Sometimes both methods proved to be possible. Thus people joining the army, who might catch tetanus once wounded, are 'actively' inoculated with anti-tetanus vaccine, just in case. On the other hand a civilian who cuts himself badly while gardening and gets soil in the wound may be given a 'passive' immunization by the doctor, to protect him from the germs which may have entered his body. The value of anti-tetanus inoculation was clearly shown during the British army's retreat to Dunkirk in 1940, through farming country

The development of drugs

Medicinal plants were known in China over five thousand years ago. One of them was *ephedra*, a coniferous plant containing the drug ephedrine, which is now used for asthma. Medicinal herbs were grown in monasteries during the Middle Ages and, as the use of medicines increased, apothecaries' shops were opened where remedies were prepared from both plants and minerals. Some of the remedies used were effective in certain circumstances, but so little was known about them that they could be dangerous if wrongly administered. It is only recently that the active principles of some remedies have been isolated as drugs, and scientifically tested for correct dosage and possible side-effects.

1618 The first *London Pharmacopoeia* published. This gave the seal of approval of the Royal College of Physicians to a list of plants and preparations.

1785 Digitalis, found in the leaves of the foxglove, first used in cases of heart disease. It is still used, but now the dosage is carefully calculated.

1803–19 Chemists began to isolate from plants various constituents which are sometimes so effective against disease, e.g. alkaloids. Three of the best known alkaloids are morphine, quinine and strychnine.

1819 Iodine used successfully in the treatment of goitre (a swelling of the thyroid gland in the neck). It was first prepared from seaweed in 1812.

1820 Isolation of quinine, the most important alkaloid in the *cinchona* bark. The cinchona plant had long been used by South American Indians as a way of reducing, if not curing, malarial fever. It was introduced to Europe in 1632 by the Jesuits and for a long time was known as Jesuits' Bark.

1876 Salicylates introduced in the treatment of rheumatism. These chemicals, found in willow and poplar trees, reduce pain and fever.

1885 Amyl nitrate first used in the treatment of angina, a heart disease. It is still used today.

1898 Barbitone first used as a sedative. It is still used today in an improved form called phenobarbitone.

1899 Aspirin first sold in a commercial form. The main pain-relieving drugs before aspirin were sedatives and narcotics such as opium, belladonna, ether and henbane.

1910 The German scientist, Paul Ehrlich, discovered the synthetic drug, salvarsan. It was the first 'magic bullet' —that is, a drug which would destroy internal infection without harming the patient. From then on, synthetic drugs began to take the place of drugs from natural sources.

1911–12 The presence of vitamins in food and their importance to health proved.

1921 Frederick Banting and Charles Best isolated insulin.

1928 Alexander Fleming discovered penicillin, but no practical use was yet made of its antibiotic effect.

1932 Prontosil, the most effective drug yet against bacterial infection, used by Gerhard Domagk to save his own daughter from blood poisoning.

1939 Paul Müller produced the pesticide, dichloro-diphenyl-trichloro-ethane, or D.D.T. Later, in 1944, it was used to check a typhus epidemic in Naples.

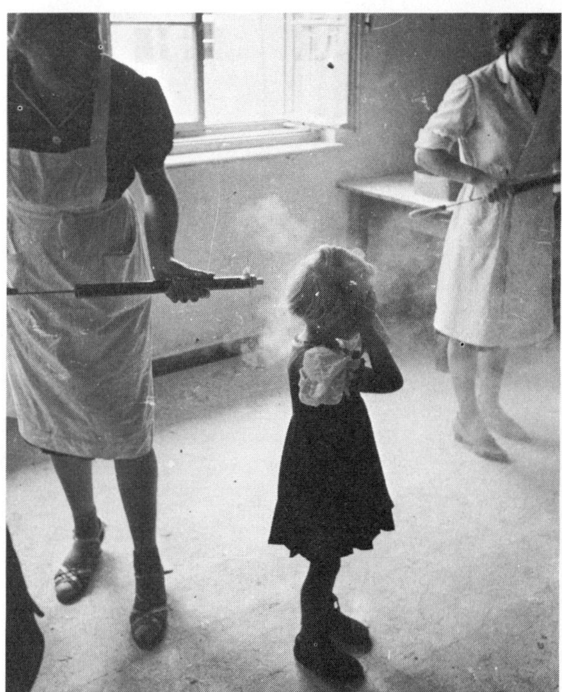

1939–40 Professor Howard Florey and Dr E. B. Chain carried out further research on penicillin in Oxford. Experiments proved its effectiveness, but supplies ran out.

1942 Penicillin began to be mass-produced in the United States.

where tetanus was known to be present in the soil. Although 16,000 men were wounded only seven cases of the disease occurred, and all among men who had refused to be inoculated against it.

Vaccines are made in two main ways, by destroying the micro-organisms and using a 'killed' vaccine to provide protection, or by deliberately weakening an organism until, though 'live', it is too weak to harm the body. Although most vaccines are injected into the bloodstream, in the last few years it has become possible for more and more to be given by mouth. Protection against polio, for instance, which a few years ago involved several injections, can now be obtained by sucking a number of lumps of sugar containing the vaccine.

Internal infection

The discovery of microbes, which transformed surgery, led to the development of immunization which revolutionized general medicine. At the same time, the coming of both anaesthetics and antiseptics led to the beginning of serious research to discover new drugs. Today, in addition to government-financed research, there is an enormous and wealthy drugs industry, which employs thousands of doctors and scientists and spends millions of pounds in the search for new and improved remedies. In 1867, when the great leap forward in medicine began, most doctors relied on a few well-tried drugs which had been in use for centuries. It was not until the last decade of the nineteenth century that many drugs were introduced which are now household words. Barbitone, now used in an improved form as phenobarbitone, began its career as a sedative, for example, in 1898, and aspirin, now the commonest of all pain-reducing remedies, in 1899. As every branch of science advanced, the doctors worked more and more closely not merely with chemists and biologists engaged in 'pure' research but with the many scientists working in industry. The outstanding need was for what was called 'a magic bullet', which would destroy internal infection, as Lister's carbolic acid destroyed external infection, without harming the patient. The first to find such a drug was a German, Paul Ehrlich, who in 1910 announced the discovery of salvarsan, a compound which was effective against the then common and often deadly disease of syphilis. (He at first called it '606', because it was the 606th compound he had tried for this purpose — a reminder of the immense amount of hard work and perseverance needed in such research.) This drug was one of a group derived from dyes and in 1932 another German, Gerhard Domagk, found that a red dye, Prontosil, was also effective against other infections. The first person to be saved by it was his own daughter, Hildegarde, who was dying of blood-poisoning after pricking herself with an infected needle in his laboratory. An improved version of the drug was used at Queen Charlotte's Maternity Hospital in London in 1935 where, despite all the advance that had been made, a few cases of puerperal fever still occurred. The use of prontosil cut the death rate of those affected from 71 to 27 per cent and later to nothing. Three years later two chemists working for a British drug firm, May and Baker, succeeded in manufacturing a new drug in the same group, at first known as 'M and B 693' because they, and the firm, had previously experimented with 692 others. After experiments on mice it was tried out for the first time in March 1938 on a Norfolk farm labourer who was dying of pneumonia; within a few days he was out of danger.

The drug, now known as sulphonamide, proved effective, too, against many other diseases, including meningitis, which attacks the brain, and osteomyelitis, which destroys the bone marrow. It was found to be useful against an annoying variety of bacteria called

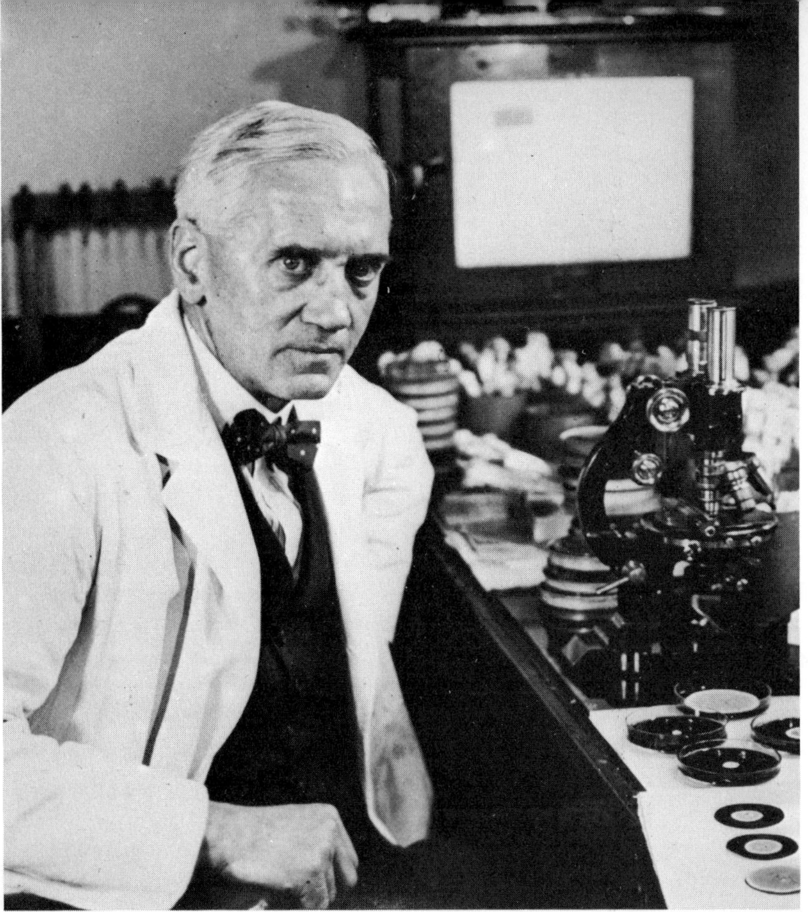

Sir Alexander Fleming who discovered the properties of the substance he named 'penicillin'.

Right Fleming's original culture plate on which he was cultivating some organisms for another purpose. The large white blob at the top was a mould which had somehow established itself on the plate. Before throwing the useless plate away, Fleming noticed something odd: this new mould seemed to kill off the organisms around it. Later, Fleming established that there were many other organisms this new mould would act against, and that 'penicillin' was not harmful to human beings.

The photograph far right shows a modern plant for manufacturing antibiotics.

staphylococcus, which often caused boils and wound infections in hospital. During the Second World War it saved thousands of lives, among them that of Britain's war-time leader, Winston Churchill. By 1942 more than 2,000 different versions of the original drug had been tried to discover which seemed 'tailor made' to attack one particular microbe. This type of experiment is an important aspect of modern pharmaceutical research. The somewhat 'hit and miss' methods of the early days of antiseptics, when all bacteria were killed indiscriminately, are long past.

The miracle drug

The sulphonamide drugs were antibiotic in their action — that is they worked by preventing the growth or multiplication of bacteria, rather than by killing them outright. Doctors had hardly realized the immense difference they had made to medicine when an even more powerful weapon was added to their armoury. The story of the discovery of penicillin is as romantic as any anecdote of Pasteur or Koch, although it involves a somewhat dour Scot, Alexander Fleming, the son of a farmer, who having left school at fifteen to work as a clerk in a London shipping office, used some money he was left by an uncle to train as a doctor. At St Mary's Hospital, Paddington, he became a pupil of Sir Almroth Wright, the pioneer of anti-typhoid inoculation, and after qualifying he remained at St Mary's. While serving four years with the Royal Army Medical Corps in France, he saw many deep wounds caused by bullets and shell fragments which led to blood-poisoning and gangrene. The ordinary antiseptics seemed powerless to halt the infection, and after the war he continued his research as a bacteriologist and pathologist — or student of diseases.

In medical matters Fleming was usually progressive;

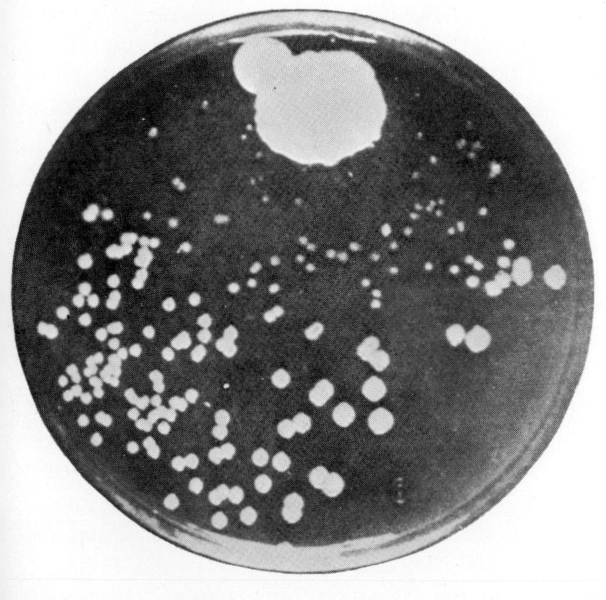

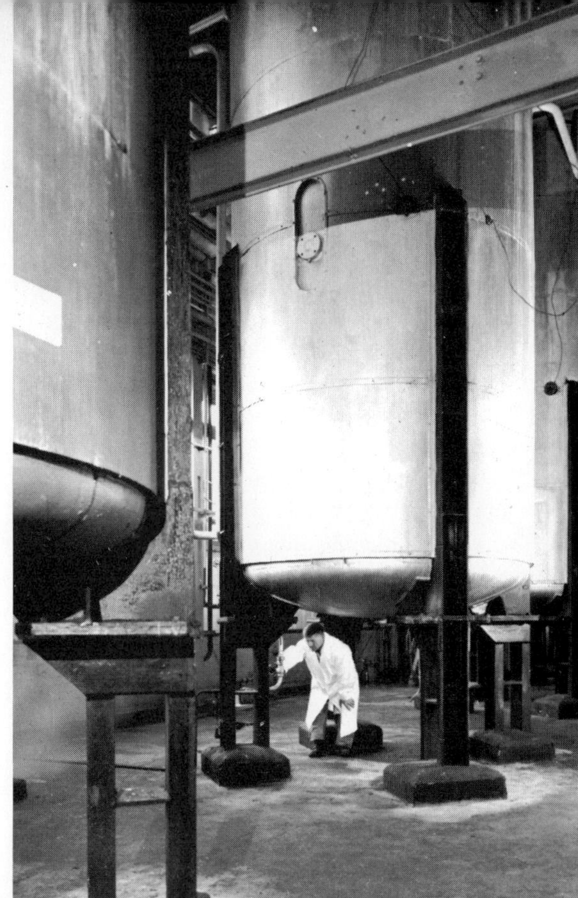

he was one of the first doctors in England to use the drug salvarsan and to make blood transfusion a regular routine, but he opposed the admission of women medical students to St Mary's and when, in 1915, he married a nurse, his friends refused to believe it until he had produced her photograph. His patients often thought him cold and distant and though he was fond of outdoor games, his life really revolved round his laboratory, where his outstanding feature as a researcher was his power of patient and persevering observation.

It was this which led him, in 1928, to note down the details when, on entering his laboratory one morning, he found that some dust which had settled on one of the dishes on his bench had started to grow a mould which, wherever it spread, had checked the growth of the bacteria being cultivated there. Pasteur had once said that 'Fortune favours the prepared mind'. Fleming realized immediately that the new mould might be useful. When, however, he tried it on a woman who was dying of blood poisoning, after a leg amputation, it failed to save her – probably because, we now know, the concentration of the drug was too weak. A chemist whom Fleming consulted, however, predicted it would be impossible to purify the mould and produce it commercially as a drug. The 'magic bullet' of the sulphonamides had just been discovered, and after publishing an account of his work on 'penicillin', as he called the drug made from the mould, Fleming turned to other work.

Then, with another war approaching, two doctors at Oxford, an Australian, Professor Howard Florey, and a German Jew, Dr E. B. Chain, read Fleming's article and, with money provided by the American Rockefeller Foundation, began serious research upon penicillin in 1939. After a long series of experiments, the moment approached for the decisive test. On 1 July 1940, fifty mice were injected with a dose of virulent streptococci, a type of bacteria, after which twenty-five of them were given penicillin every three hours, for two days and nights. At the end of sixteen hours the scientists knew they had made a great discovery: all the twenty-five mice who had not been given penicillin were dead; but only one of those who *had* been injected with it.

To produce enough penicillin for practical use proved enormously difficult. The first patient on whom it was tried, a policeman dying of blood poisoning whom the sulphonamides had failed to help, showed a miraculous improvement, but supplies of the drug ran out and he died. Then, in April 1941, came two successful cases, a fifteen year old boy with an infected hip wound, and another patient suffering from a huge carbuncle. With only this evidence to support his claims, Florey went to America to find a firm which would produce the drug – British factories were now fully stretched with war work and under bombing attack.

But the American drug industry, once convinced that this was indeed 'the miracle drug' for which doctors had been searching for nearly a century, tackled the job of producing it on a large scale with characteristic energy. In 1942 they produced only enough to treat fifteen wounded soldiers in the whole of the British Eighth Army in Egypt. By 1944 penicillin was in use on every battle front and in every civilian hospital where doctors could obtain the precious supplies. Not merely did it enable military casualties to be returned quickly to duty, but it prevented complications developing in the hand injuries common among workers in the war factories. Penicillin was at this time extremely expensive, but in wartime this was a secondary matter. A Scottish scientific writer later recalled how:

Towards the end of the war I was in hospital being treated for generalized septicaemia [blood-poisoning]. I had a hollow needle in my leg and penicillin was being dripped into it. I knew the cost of the product. It was a Scotsman's nightmare. I lay there and counted each drip. 'Tenpence. Tenpence. Tenpence . . .'.

Fortunately mass production soon brought the price down and now the glass ampoule containing each dose costs more than the drug it contains.

By 1945, when the war ended, the United States was producing twenty times as much penicillin as Britain and the manufacture of the drug had become big business on both sides of the Atlantic. Some of the American scientists who perfected the manufacturing process took out patents on their work, so they receive a payment from anyone who uses it, but the British doctors who had made the first discoveries never patented their work. Had they done so their patents might by now have earned millions of pounds for themselves and for Great Britain. However, they were rewarded in other ways; Fleming and Florey were both knighted and later, with Dr Chain, were jointly awarded the great honour of the Nobel Prize for Medicine.

Today penicillin is used in every hospital and prescribed by every doctor. Cuts and wounds are often packed with penicillin powder, to stop the harmful bacteria multiplying, and it is used on burns, abscesses and skin infections, and to prevent complications developing in minor ailments of, say, the ear or throat. Its outstanding contribution has been, however, within the body against such persistent enemies as blood-poisoning, meningitis, pneumonia and venereal disease, where it has largely replaced the first 'magic bullet', salvarsan. In some cases, like osteomyelitis, an inflammation of the bone marrow which particularly attacks children, penicillin has not merely drastically reduced the death rate but has often made major surgery unnecessary.

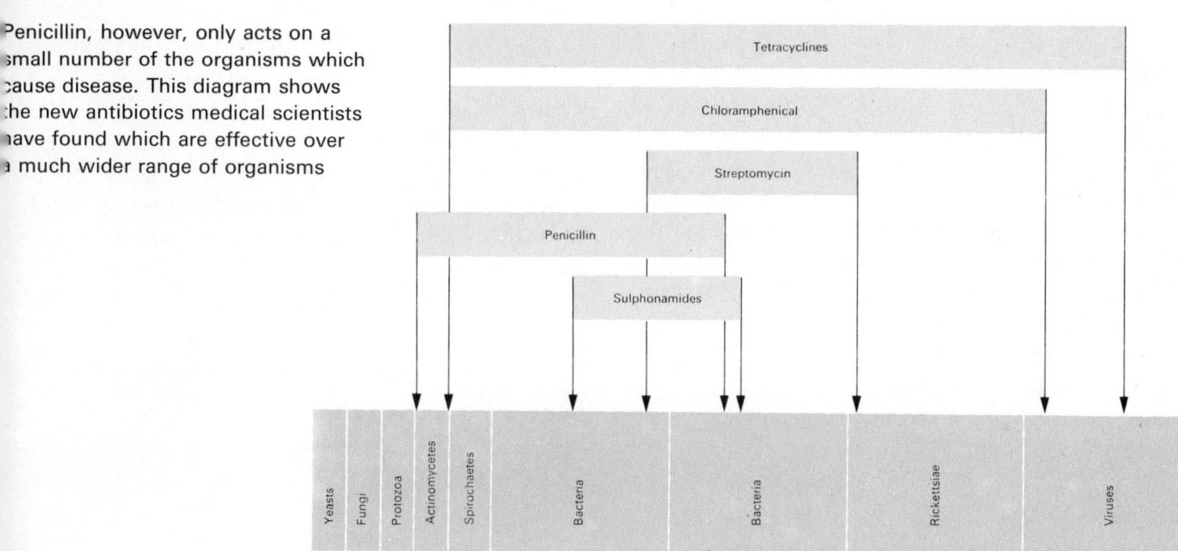

Penicillin, however, only acts on a small number of the organisms which cause disease. This diagram shows the new antibiotics medical scientists have found which are effective over a much wider range of organisms

Disease without germs

Although this book has dealt mainly with infectious diseases caused and spread by germs, there are, of course, many other diseases which attack an individual's body for reasons we do not really understand. Disorders may begin in a particular gland, or in the structure of the tiny cells of which the bone and flesh and blood are composed. Such diseases cannot be halted by preventive medicine or immunization in the way that cholera or diphtheria or tuberculosis have been checked. Often they cannot be cured, though they can be treated.

A good example of such a disease is diabetes, which has puzzled doctors since at least 2,000 B.C. People suffering from the disease used to feel permanently tired, to lose weight however much they ate and finally took to their beds, sank into a coma and died. The disease was a cruel one for the patient, who became each week a little thinner and weaker, and who could be kept alive only on a strict diet that excluded all forms of starch and sugar, so that bread, jam, puddings and soft drinks were all forbidden. For the doctor, diabetes was intensely frustrating for, though he knew what was wrong, he had no idea how to set it right.

The first step forward came only in 1899, when a German doctor proved that the seat of the disease was the pancreas, a small organ situated behind the stomach. The next step came a few years later in Toronto, where in 1919 a young Canadian doctor, Frederick Banting, first began actively to study the disease. Banting, a farmer's son, had been deeply upset as a child when a girl of his own age died of diabetes and as a young man he gave up studying to become a Methodist minister to read medicine instead. After qualifying as a surgeon in the Army during the First World War, he set up as a specialist in orthopaedics, but patients were not numerous and he had ample spare-time. He began to read about diabetes and in the summer of 1921 he managed to borrow a laboratory from a Scottish professor at the university who was going home for a holiday. A twenty-one year old medical student, Charles Best, the son of a country doctor, offered to spend his vacation helping Banting with his research.

All through the long, scorchingly hot, summer days the two young men slaved away in their small, bare laboratory and in the attic room where they kept the dogs on which they were experimenting. They had no help and little money; whatever had to be done they did themselves — feeding the dogs, collecting samples of their urine, cleaning up after them. Often they slept in the laboratory, waking every two hours to make observations and carry out tests, and when they ran out of funds Banting sold his car to keep the research going.

By the end of the year Banting and Best had proved that the reason people suffered from diabetes was that their pancreas failed to produce a vital substance which enabled their blood to absorb sugar. Instead it passed out of their body unused, however much they ate, until they virtually starved to death. More important still, they had succeeded in making the missing substance, later called 'insulin', from healthy pancreases, first of dogs and then of cows.

In January 1922 the new drug was for the first time tried on a human patient, a boy of eleven, who weighed only sixty-five pounds and who, when the risks were explained to him, replied, 'Yes, I should like to have it.' Within a few weeks he was putting on weight; soon he was able to live a normal life.

Few drugs have been discovered or brought into use so rapidly as insulin, for within a few months it was being presented all over the world. Within four years Banting had been knighted and he and Best had been given the Nobel Prize for Medicine. Best, after finishing his medical training, moved on to new research. Banting, while flying to England to conduct experiments to help airmen, was killed in an air crash in 1941. Today there are about 300,000 known diabetics in Great Britain, each of whom, provided he injects himself with insulin and watches his diet, can lead an otherwise normal life. Three hundred thousand more people are believed to have the disease without yet realizing it. Once all these would have faced a death sentence; now, thanks to the work of two men, they should, barring accidents, live to old age.

Banting and Best, discoverers of insulin, and a healthy enough dog.

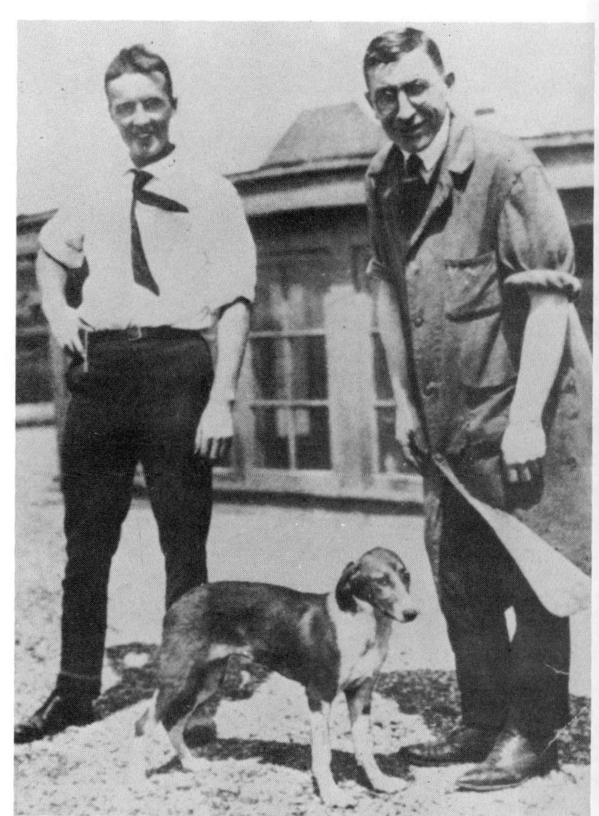

The control of epidemic diseases

Until a hundred years ago overcrowding, dirt, bad sanitation and ignorance meant that nothing could stop the spread of an epidemic. The most terrifying was probably the Black Death, a form of plague carried by flea-infested rats. It struck Europe in the fourteenth century when about a quarter of the total population died in a cycle of epidemics. People imagined the Black Death as a man on a black horse, or else as a black giant striding along, his head above the rooftops. In the fifteenth, sixteenth and seventeenth centuries there were at least thirteen major epidemics in England alone. The epidemic in 1665 was the last English epidemic, but not the last European one for Messina lost 70,000 inhabitants in an outbreak in 1743 (though a further outbreak was recorded in Cyprus in 1759).

When cholera began to spread from India across the world in 1821, people must have been reminded of the Black Death which had lingered in street-songs and popular legend, but it was soon realized that the Asiatic cholera was an entirely new disease.

1701 An Italian doctor inoculated three children in Constantinople with the smallpox virus which gave them immunity against the disease.

1718 Lady Mary Wortley Montagu introduced inoculation to Britain having seen how effective it was in Turkey. The method continued to be used from time to time, arousing as much opposition as support.

1796 Edward Jenner successfully carried out his first experiment in vaccination against smallpox on an eight-year-old boy. After that, this new preventive measure using a cowpox virus rapidly spread to other countries.

1831–33 First cholera epidemic in Britain. About 60,000 people died.

1848–49 Second cholera epidemic. Nearly half a million people died.

1849 John Snow's book, *On the Mode of Communication of Cholera*, suggested a link between infection and a contaminated water supply.

1853 Vaccination against smallpox made compulsory in Britain.

1861 Semmelweiss, a Hungarian doctor, published the result of his work on puerperal ('childbed') fever.

1864 Louis Pasteur proved that infections are caused by micro-organisms.

1866 Last great cholera epidemic in Britain.

1882 Robert Koch isolated the bacterium responsible for tuberculosis. Two years later he isolated the cholera bacterium.

1890 Pasteur successfully inoculated patients against rabies, a fatal disease caused by the bite of a mad dog.

1894 New diptheria anti-toxin tried out in Paris. It greatly reduced the death rate from this disease.

1896 Sir Almroth Wright carried out the first anti-typhoid vaccination.

1897 It was proved in Japan that bubonic plague is carried by flea-infested rats.
Sir Ronald Ross discovered that the mosquito is responsible for transmitting malaria.

1901 Yellow fever virus identified. An American team eradicated yellow fever from Havana, Cuba, by spraying the undergrowth in the mosquito breeding grounds with burning petrol, by scattering sand in the holes in the sea-shore to prevent mosquitoes breeding in the sea-water, and by destroying insanitary housing.

1905 First successful anti-cholera vaccine produced in India.

1906 Vaccine against bubonic plague first used in India.

1908 Polio virus isolated by Karl Landsteiner.

1914 Large-scale anti-cholera vaccination introduced.

1918–19 World-wide influenza epidemic in which approximately twenty million people died.
Various vaccines were tried out in the United States between 1942 and the Asian flu epidemic of 1957 with some success, but no vaccine yet discovered is entirely effective against all strains of flu.

1928 First yellow-fever vaccine produced.

1938 Ministry of Health launched a campaign to persuade people to have their children immunized against diptheria. Dramatic decline in deaths from diptheria after this.

1954 First mass trial of Jonas Salk's anti-polio vaccine was successful.

1964 Aberdeen typhoid epidemic successfully contained without mass immunization. No deaths.

1965 Vaccine against ordinary measles introduced in Britain, though no effective programme came into operation until 1967.

1969 Vaccine against German measles under trial by the Medical Research Council.

7 Doctors and statesmen

Medical progress was enthusiastically welcomed by those who could afford to call in a doctor. But a large section of the population — up to 28 per cent in the towns and cities — seldom earned enough money to buy essential food and clothing let alone pay for the services of a G.P. For these slum dwellers, illness and sudden death were not at all unusual, but even the better paid workers relied heavily on private charities or the generosity of individual doctors for any medical treatment they might need.

Some of them paid regular weekly contributions into insurance schemes run by trade unions and clubs so that they could obtain free medical advice in an emergency. At the beginning of this century many social reformers believed that the government should take over this idea and operate an insurance scheme to cover all those who could not afford to go to hospital or visit a surgery. The suggestion attracted the interest of David Lloyd George, a Liberal politician who was Chancellor of the Exchequer from 1908 to 1915 and Prime Minister during the First World War. His Welsh parents had known what it was like to be short of money and his father died of tuberculosis. Moreover, the country was in the mood for social reform and the Liberal Government had introduced a number of measures, including old age pensions, to make life a little easier for the poorer members of the community.

The National Insurance Act was approved by Parliament in 1911. One section of the new law dealt with the problem of unemployment in trades where workers were liable to lose their jobs without any notice. Small sums of money were paid out to tide them over until they were able to find other employment. But the section of the Act dealing with health insurance covered all wage-earners drawing less than £3 a week — then a fair income for, say, a railway worker or a clerk. Each member of the scheme paid fourpence a week; his employer added threepence and the government twopence — hence the slogan 'ninepence for fourpence'. In return, ten shillings a week was paid to any man who was off work because of sickness and he could call on a doctor to treat him free of charge. Wives and children were not included in the plan and the payments were certainly not very generous. Even so, the Act aroused a good deal of opposition, particularly from doctors who did not like the idea of government control.

Two pieces of propaganda for Lloyd George in the 1911 election. The one below comes from a poster captioned 'The Right Ticket for You! You are Travelling on a Safe Line and are Assured of a Safe Return'. Right is a postcard reproducing the insurance stamp. It was around this time that many of the techniques of modern advertising first began to be used. Lord Kitchener's famous recruiting posters for the First World War were only a few years away.

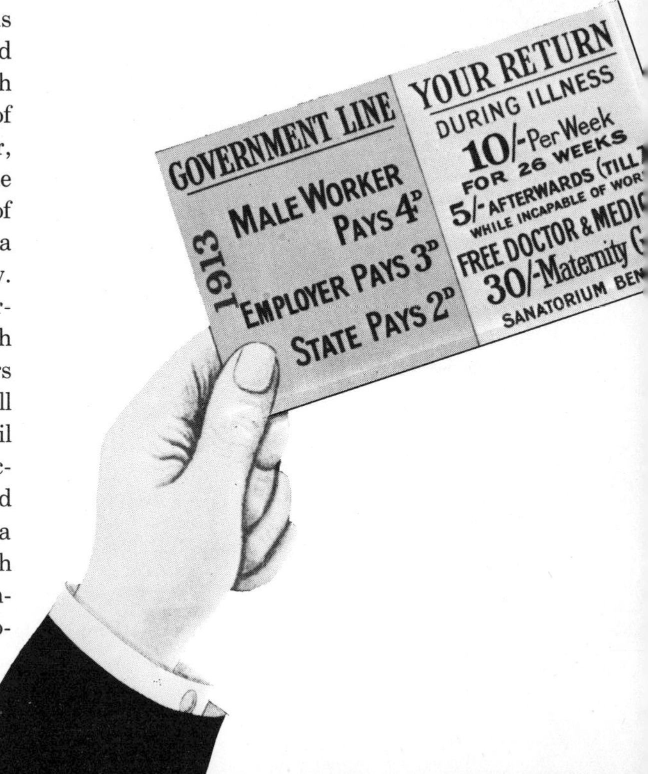

Lloyd George had to work hard to win their approval and he only succeeded by agreeing to their financial demands. Doctors who prescribed for poor people or 'panel' patients were able to rely on a good regular income for their services.

Employers regarded the Act as an additional tax burden and a nuisance because each week their office clerks had to stick insurance stamps into the cards of every one of their workers. Titled ladies boasted they would 'never lick stamps for Mr Lloyd George', and *The Times* went so far as to advise its readers to defy the law. No wonder Lloyd George was heard to say, 'Never was legislation more needed. Never was it less wanted.'

THE STAMP THAT WANTS
A LOT OF LICKING
AND THE MAN

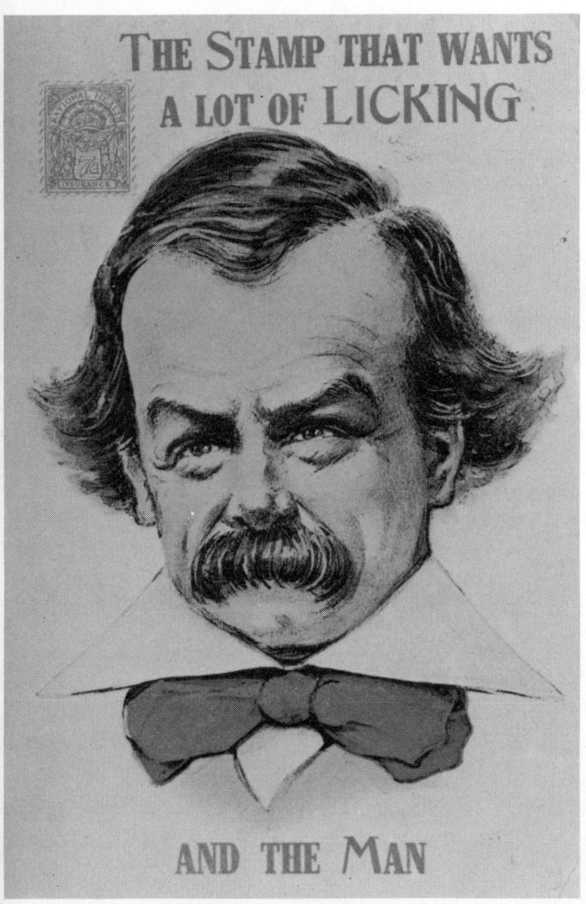

Improvements in the health services were also taking place at a local level. One of the chief worries of the medical experts was the high infant mortality rate — in 1899, 163 out of every thousand babies died during their first year.

In poor districts the percentage was much higher than in the better off areas and some of the more advanced town councils started to organize the provision of milk and offer advice to mothers on how to look after their children. Then the government stepped in and granted financial help for the building of maternity hospitals and infant welfare centres or 'schools for mothers' as they were known at the time. The battle against ignorance and poverty achieved a reduction in the infant mortality rate from 151 in every thousand in 1901, to 128 in 1905 and ninety-five in 1912. After 1906, older children were able to buy cheap school meals and medical examinations were arranged so that doctors could advise the parents if their families needed treatment.

There was a limit to what could be done in the way of preventing illness and disease without raising general living standards. This meant building more houses, improving sanitation and, above all, providing everyone with a decent wage. The point was made very clear in 1918, when it was discovered that an average of only three in nine men who signed on for the army were fit and healthy. Conditions changed for the better as the country became wealthier, but meanwhile attempts were made to make the health services more efficient.

The Ministry of Health was set up in 1919. Before

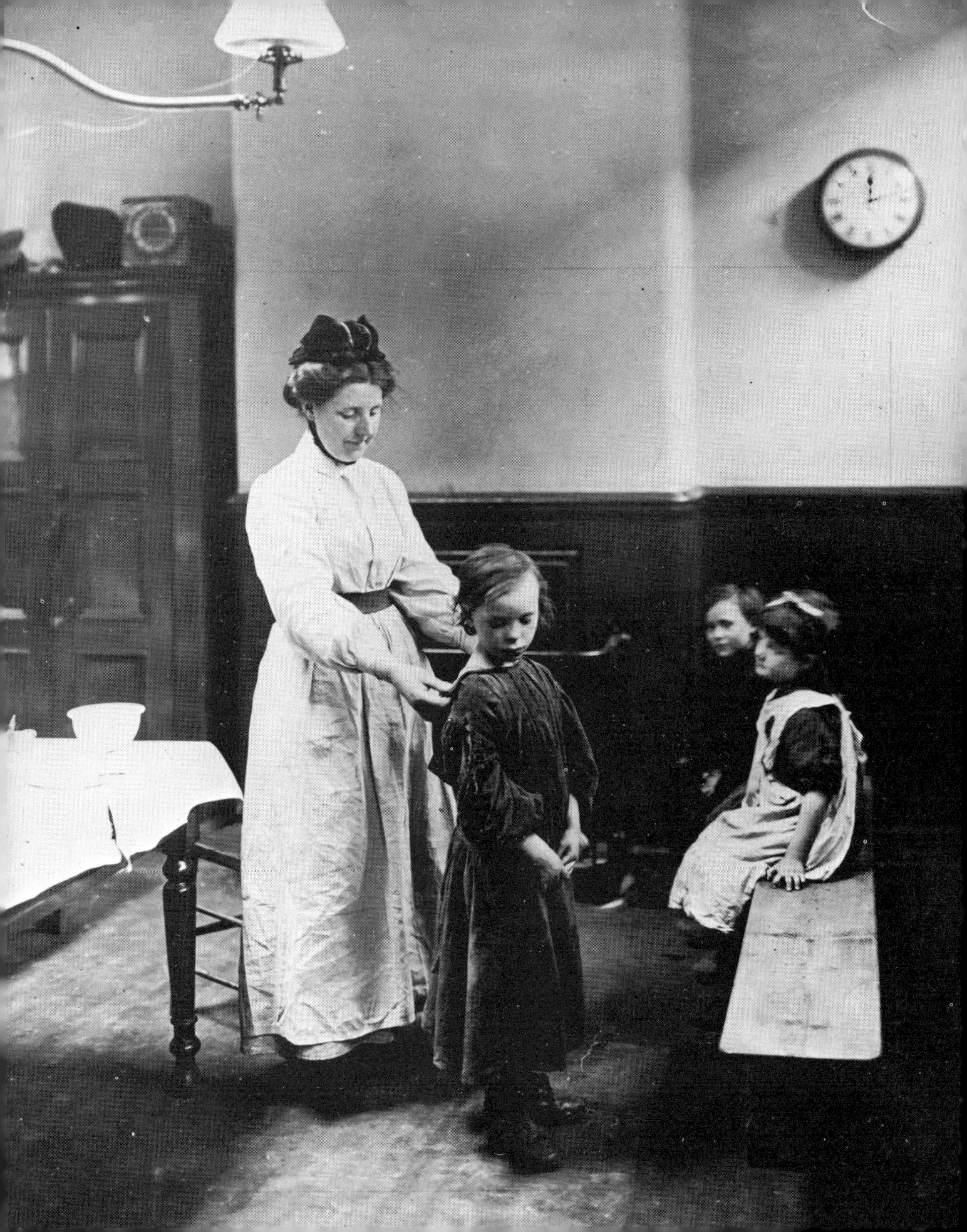

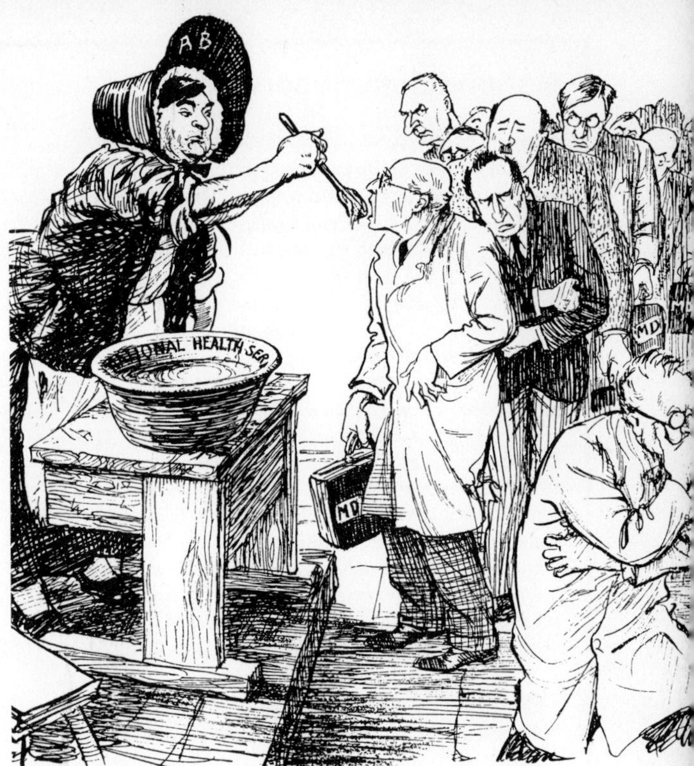

Left A 'cleansing station' in 1912. Most of the medical and social workers came from the educated middle class, and it was difficult for them to conceal their distaste for the insanitary conditions of the people they worked among. Not unnaturally, many poor people felt uncomfortable in this situation, and avoided treatment when they could.

Right In this cartoon from *Punch* in 1948, Aneurin Bevan, Minister of Health in the Labour Government, is shown dishing out very bitter medicine to the country's doctors.

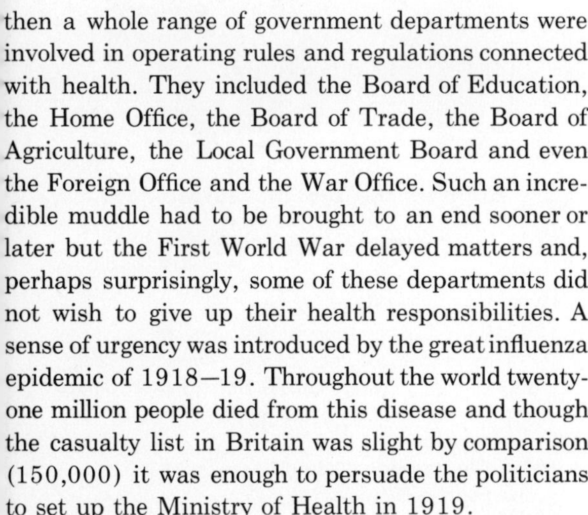

then a whole range of government departments were involved in operating rules and regulations connected with health. They included the Board of Education, the Home Office, the Board of Trade, the Board of Agriculture, the Local Government Board and even the Foreign Office and the War Office. Such an incredible muddle had to be brought to an end sooner or later but the First World War delayed matters and, perhaps surprisingly, some of these departments did not wish to give up their health responsibilities. A sense of urgency was introduced by the great influenza epidemic of 1918–19. Throughout the world twenty-one million people died from this disease and though the casualty list in Britain was slight by comparison (150,000) it was enough to persuade the politicians to set up the Ministry of Health in 1919.

In the period between the two World Wars the number of people covered by health insurance almost doubled, but still only half the population were in the scheme. The rest had to wait until 1948, when Aneurin Bevan, Labour Minister of Health and a Welshman, introduced the National Health Service. This system, designed to improve and maintain the health of everyone in the country, was originally 'free' to all users. That is, it was paid for partly from taxes and partly from the weekly subscription, in the form of stamps on a card, shared by employer and employee. A patient could then make use of a wide range of facilities without paying at the time of treatment. Nowadays, (unless he is excused payment for some special reason, for example, old age) he has to pay a small charge for such things as spectacles, hearing aids, false teeth and dental treatment, and medicines obtained on prescription. But he can still visit his doctor, and through him obtain essential hospital care, surgery or specialist treatment, all without further payment.

This is the 'curing' side of the National Health Service, but there are also large sections of it devoted to preventing disease and caring for particular groups of the community such as the very young, the old, the disabled, and expectant mothers. It also provides money for research and controls the quality and safety

National health services

National health services are not a new invention. In Ancient Greece communities often paid physicians an annual salary raised from taxes. The Romans organized a public medical service in the second century A.D., in which public physicians gave medical treatment to the poor in return for a salary paid by the city or town.

In Britain the idea of a state-run health service was discussed in books long before it became actual fact. Sir Thomas More worked out a complicated plan in his book, *Utopia*, published in 1524.

Daniel Defoe, in the early eighteen century, thought that insurance should be used to finance medical treatment for the poor. In fact, by 1810, there were more than 7,000 'friendly societies' in England and Wales working on this principle. On the Continent, it was Germany who set the example for national medical care. Hamburg, for example, financed it from taxation and voluntary contributions.

1793 The Friendly Societies Act provided legal status and protection for the funds of these societies.

1779 An Austrian professor, Johann Frank, thought it the duty of the state to supervise health at all times, not only during epidemics. His book, *System of Medical Police*, laid down the principles of a state health service. These principles were put into practice in France during the Napoleonic period and in certain German states.

1795 Manchester Board of Health formed following a series of typhus epidemics.

1805 A central Board of Health formed in London in the face of a threat of yellow fever spreading from the Mediterranean, but it was disbanded after eighteen months.

1831 Boards of Health appointed in 1,200 districts in Britain because of the cholera epidemic.

1834 Report of the Royal Commission on the Poor Law set up medical officers in the Poor Law Unions and central inspectors in London.

1848 Public Health Act established a national Board of Health with the power to establish local Boards of Health when asked by not less than one tenth of the ratepayers.

1858 The Privy Council took over the function of the national Board of Health until 1871, when the Local Government Board took its place.

1861 Russia set up the *Zemstvo* system, under which the country was divided into regions, each with its salaried doctors and hospital building programme.

1883 Bismarck set up a social insurance scheme in Prussia. Based on schemes already operating in certain German states, it was soon copied in Austria (1888), Hungary (1891), Luxembourg (1901), Norway (1909) and Switzerland (1911).

1911 Lloyd George introduced the first national insurance schemes including the 'ninepence for fourpence' system for free medical treatment. The scheme only applied to the worker who paid his contribution, and not to his wife and children.

THE DAWN OF HOPE.

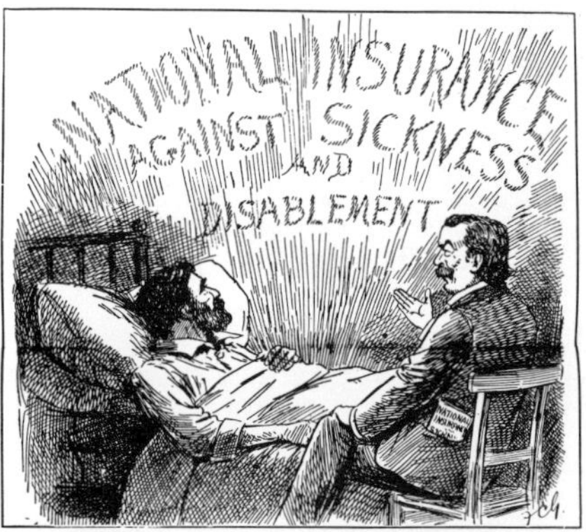

Mr. LLOYD GEORGE'S National Health Insurance Bill provides for the insurance of the Worker in case of Sickness.

Support the Liberal Government
in their policy of
SOCIAL REFORM.

1919 Ministry of Health created.

1942 Report of the Beveridge Committee recommended a comprehensive national health service for '. . . every citizen without exceptions, without remuneration limit and without an economic barrier'.

1948 The National Health Service came into operation in Britain.

1965 President Johnson introduced Medicare in the United States: a national scheme for providing old people with free medical care. It was, in fact, first introduced by President Kennedy, but he had been unable to get the bill through Congress.

of commercially produced drugs. In the year 1966–7, Britain spent over £1,500 million on running this elaborate service, compared with £400 million in 1948, its first year of operation. Then, oddly enough, just as in 1911, the official leaders of the medical profession vowed that they would not work the scheme, they then changed their minds. Any disagreement since then has centred on how the Service should be run rather than on whether it should exist. The introduction of charges for various items has been, and still is, the subject of bitter political argument. But few people, in or out of the medical profession, would deny that the present system is far better than anything which went before. Some Western countries, however, still rely on private insurance schemes and feel that this is the best method. Perhaps, simply because health is so important, very few people are prepared to try anything new.

Public health and Aberdeen

In public health, too, the modern state has created a system capable of dealing with even quite serious outbreaks. The Aberdeen typhoid epidemic of 1964 shows how modern medicine copes with an epidemic. As soon as the disease had been positively identified by bacteriological tests on the first patients, the local Medical Officer of Health, Dr I. A. G. MacQueen, set up a team of doctors and sanitary inspectors who worked non-stop to try to trace the source and any contacts with it. Within four days there were forty-eight confirmed cases in hospital and it was obvious that the city had a major epidemic on its hands. The source of infection meanwhile had been identified as a seven pound tin of corned beef in a local shop which had contaminated a slicing machine used for other cold meats. As the number of cases grew alarmingly over the next few days, Dr MacQueen and his hard-pressed staff took various steps to try to contain the epidemic. A special hospital was taken over to house the typhoid patients and a list of their names and addresses was circulated. Anybody who had had food or drink prepared or handled by any of these 'contacts' was advised to consult his doctor immediately. Schools, clubs and dance halls in the city were closed and the citizens were asked to cancel their holidays and stay in the city. Some people criticized Dr MacQueen for not organizing mass immunization, but he pointed out that immunization would take six or seven weeks to be effective. Even then, since typhoid is a disease which has an incubation period of about twelve days before it shows itself, it would only work if the person concerned had not already been infected. He also stressed that, as the disease was not highly infectious and only communicated by direct contact, the best way to stop it spreading was strict personal hygiene. A great publicity campaign was organized to remind people of the vital necessity to wash their hands after using the lavatory or before preparing food. Forty-five thousand copies of a pamphlet called *How to Stamp Out Typhoid* were distributed, and a Scottish member of the government was photographed washing *his* hands to help drive the message home.

The government later set up an independent inquiry into the cause of the epidemic which revealed that the corned beef had probably become infected when a tin with faulty seams had been cooled in unchlorinated water at a South American packing station. A government inspector had reported these conditions at the plant, but not before some of the meat had been unloaded and circulated in Britain. When cholera reached nineteenth-century Britain there was neither the knowledge nor the organization to cope with it. Aberdeen could consider itself fortunate to have had both. Great Britain could claim, perhaps, to have washed its hands of typhoid.

Aberdeen: diary of an epidemic

Tuesday, 9 May 1964 Four patients admitted to the city hospital: uncertain diagnosis.

Wednesday, 20 May 1964 Typhoid confirmed. The Aberdeen Medical Officer of Health, Dr Ian MacQueen, organizes the long questioning of patients. Where have they been during the last few weeks? Exactly what have they eaten? Where? Who did they eat it with? The information is collected fast and analysed. Late on Wednesday evening, the first suspects: ice-cream and cold meat. Health visitors and medical officers under control of Dr MacQueen are retracing the steps of patients and their contacts.

Thursday, 21 May 1964 In the morning, ice-cream is ruled out. Centre of infection is narrowed down to three shops. By the afternoon, these three suspects have been reduced to one, and examination shows no carriers and no remaining germs.

Friday, 22 May 1964 Nearly all cases are narrowed down to corned beef from one large tin. Health Department accepts corned beef as source of outbreak. MacQueen drafts letter to the town's eighty-six General Practitioners, telling them of the presumed source. Already working all out under him are four Health Education Officers, fifteen Medical Officers, seventy-two Health Visitors and ten Sanitary Inspectors.

Saturday, 23 May 1964 The Colindale Public Health Laboratory phones from London: the bacterium is of a kind called Phage 34, which is only found in Spain, Latin America and southern United States. This clinched it: the germ was contained in a large tin of corned beef imported form Argentina. By this time there are forty-eight confirmed cases in City Hospital wards.

Monday, 25 May 1964 Sudden appearance of extra cases without corned beef history. Investigation shows that slicing machine used for corned beef had infected other sliced meats. So now there were thousands of possible cases. Three steps taken: (1) appeal to former nurses to return hospital to help; (2) massive campaign for perfect food hygiene by television, sound radio, leaflet an brochure; (3) daily meetings of heads of all service in MacQueen's office.

Thursday, 28 May 1964 MacQueen estimates th there are about 1,000 contacts of actual cases in Aberdeen, all already questioned and re-questione but 10,000 people bought cold meat from the sho between 6 and 23 May. Some of these will be developing typhoid and there is no way of identify them in advance. The City Hospital Laboratory is working overtime, doctors queuing with samples.

Friday, 29 May 1964 At his twice-daily Press Conference, MacQueen is relaxed. Doctors and health visitors are very tired, but the epidemic see to be coming under control. Almost immediately someone hands him a piece of paper. MacQueen leaves the room and returns a few minutes later: 'I have just been told that twenty-nine cases have been admitted to the hospitals since 2.30 this afternoon. Twenty-nine in the space of three hours The second phase of the epidemic had reached a new peak.

Monday, 1 June 1964 Sixty-four new cases admitted to hospital — the largest number in twen four hours since the epidemic began. As a precaution against secondary cases (infected from food handled by primary cases) MacQueen closes schools, cinemas, dance halls and bingo halls. He advises that, until the outbreak is controlled, peopl planning a holiday in Aberdeen should postpone it, and that people should only come to the town if they absolutely need to. Television and radio statements about danger of pre-cooked food and the vital necessity for hand-washing after using t lavatory rise to three or four daily.

Tuesday, 2 June 1964 The Government withdraw all tins of corned beef produced by suspect firms.

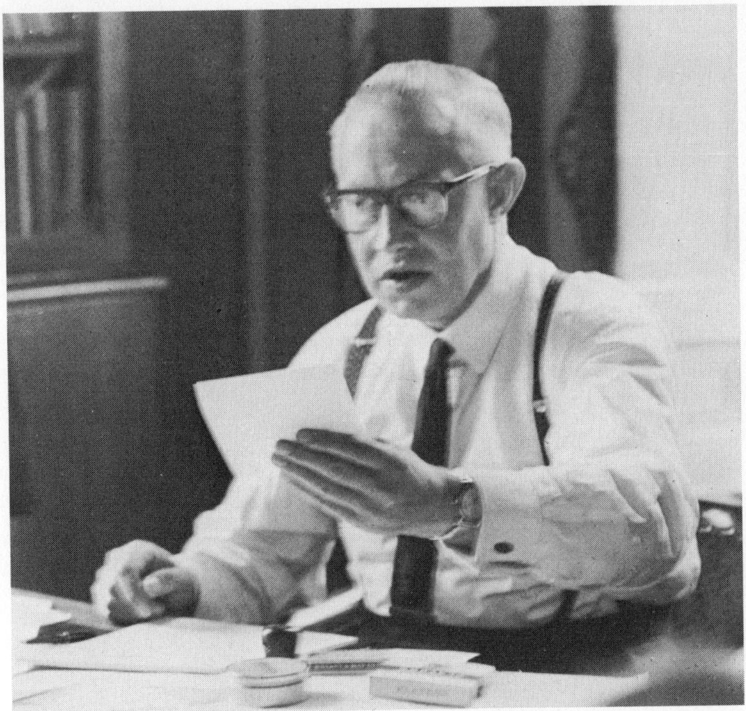

luite by chance, the camera has aught one of the most dramatic noments of the epidemic. On Friday, 9 May, Dr MacQueen begins his ress conference. Things are going vell and MacQueen seems relaxed. member of his staff enters and ands him a small piece of paper: he second wave of the epidemic as begun.

Vednesday, 3 June 1964 Cases still continue at ibout thirty a day but all from the same source: no resh centres of infection. MacQueen, now more elaxed, describes to the Press his two earlier noments of despair: the school which said that ndividual towels were an unnecessary expense which led to his closing all schools) and the woman vho, ignoring all advice about dangers of pre-cooked ood, came to complain about a pre-cooked chicken being mouldy.

Friday, 5 June 1964 New cases down to seventeen. Medical Officer of Health hints cautiously that the outbreak appears to be under control but repeats need for careful hygiene when handling food.

Monday, 8 June 1964 New cases down to ten – the lowest since the outbreak got under way. A butcher's shop is closed and £400 worth of meat destroyed.

Tuesday, 9 June 1964 Four cases. A fruit shop is closed. MacQueen's forceful pleas begin to backfire: Aberdeen people are widely regarded as 'lepers'.

Wednesday, 10 June 1964 Fifteen cases.

Tuesday, 17 June 1964 MacQueen reports to Corporation that the outbreak is controlled and the danger over. The Lord Provost's Committee votes another £15,000 to revive Aberdeen as a holiday resort.

Thursday, 18 June 1964 No more cases admitted to hospital. The restrictions are lifted.

Sunday, 28 June 1964 The Queen visits Aberdeen to demonstrate that city is really free from infection.

There have been over 400 primary cases, from corned beef and from cold meat infected by the slicing machine, and no secondary cases.

Epilogue

This book has not been a complete and comprehensive history of medicine and public health. In the space available it could hardly have been that. Instead, it has tried to show how things were before the dramatic progress of the nineteenth and twentieth centuries, and how these changes came about.

If one compares the world of medicine and public health today with that of one hundred or even thirty years ago, it is easy to feel that the progress has been so enormous that little remains to be done. Easy but wrong. In the following pages we look at some of the problems still left to be solved, and at some of the problems which the modern world has actually created.

Today about one family in four – four and a half million families altogether – live in council houses. But there are still slums and still much sub-standard housing. There are few families today without their own water tap, but one family in six still lacks its own bath. Many, too, have no lavatory inside the house.

Many public lavatories have hardly been improved since they were built, up to fifty years ago. Councils are working hard on the problem, but it is still not taken for granted that a lavatory should have facilities for washing hands. This is even true of many schools, where of all places conditions should be better.

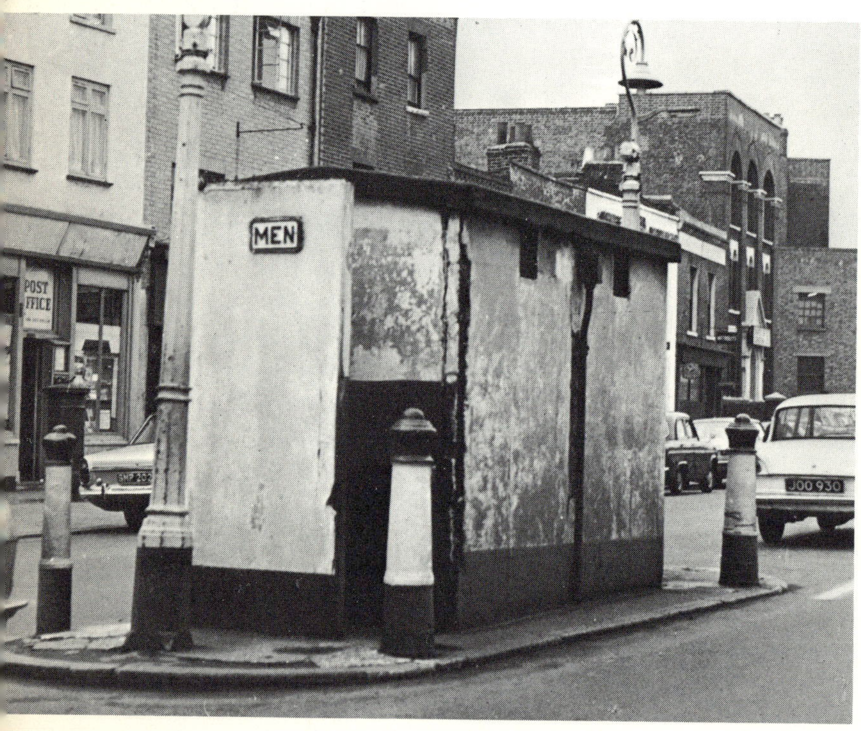

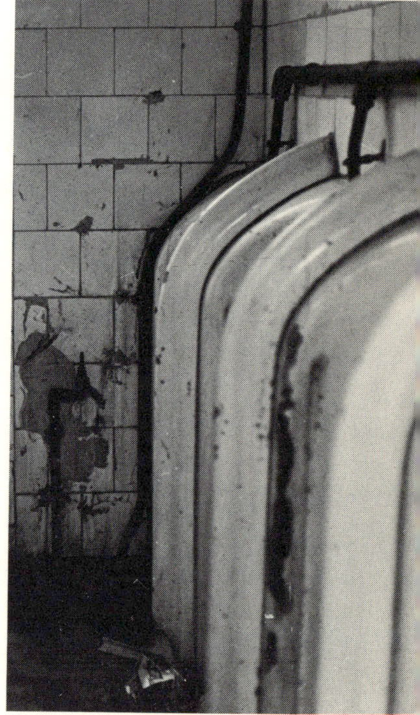

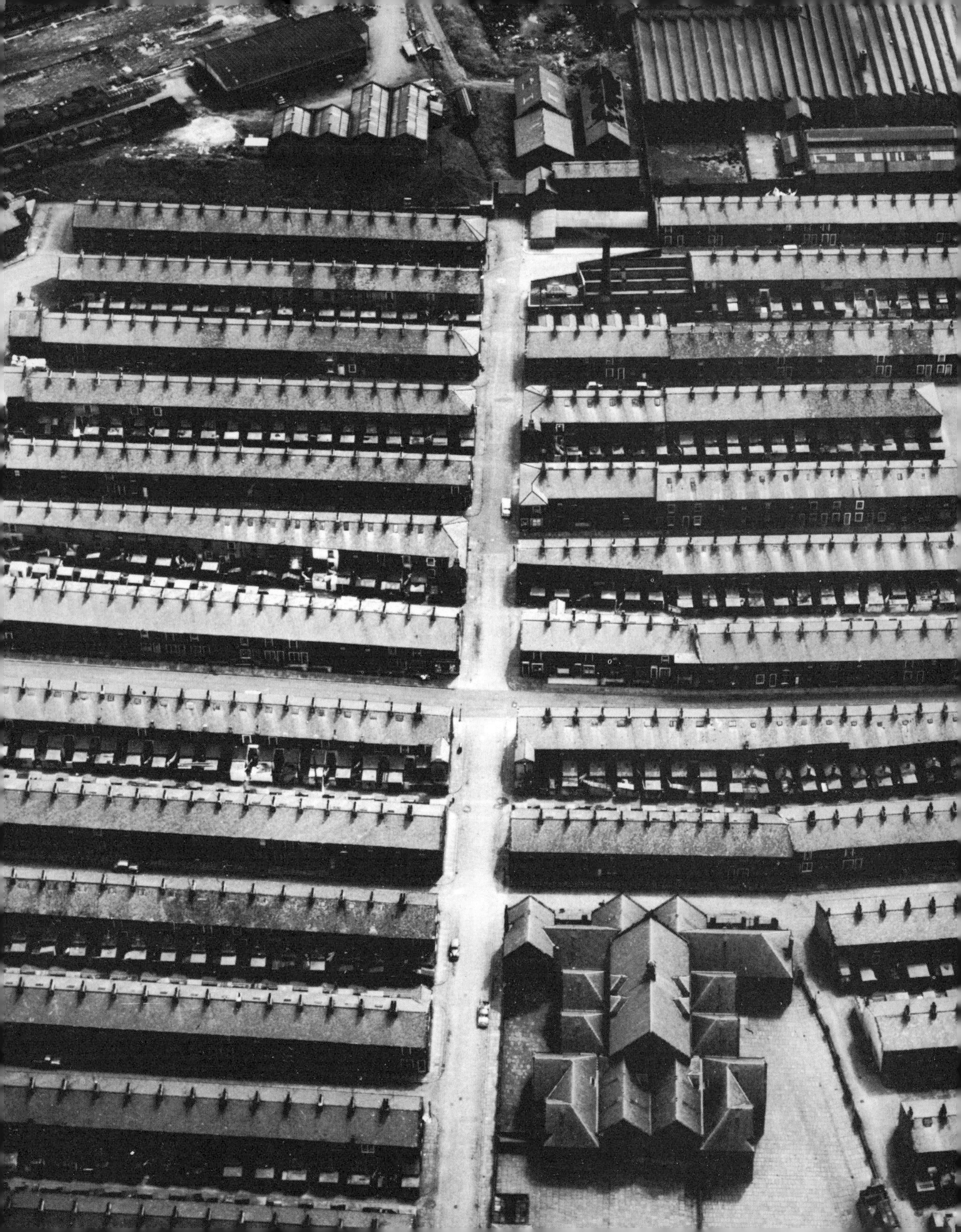

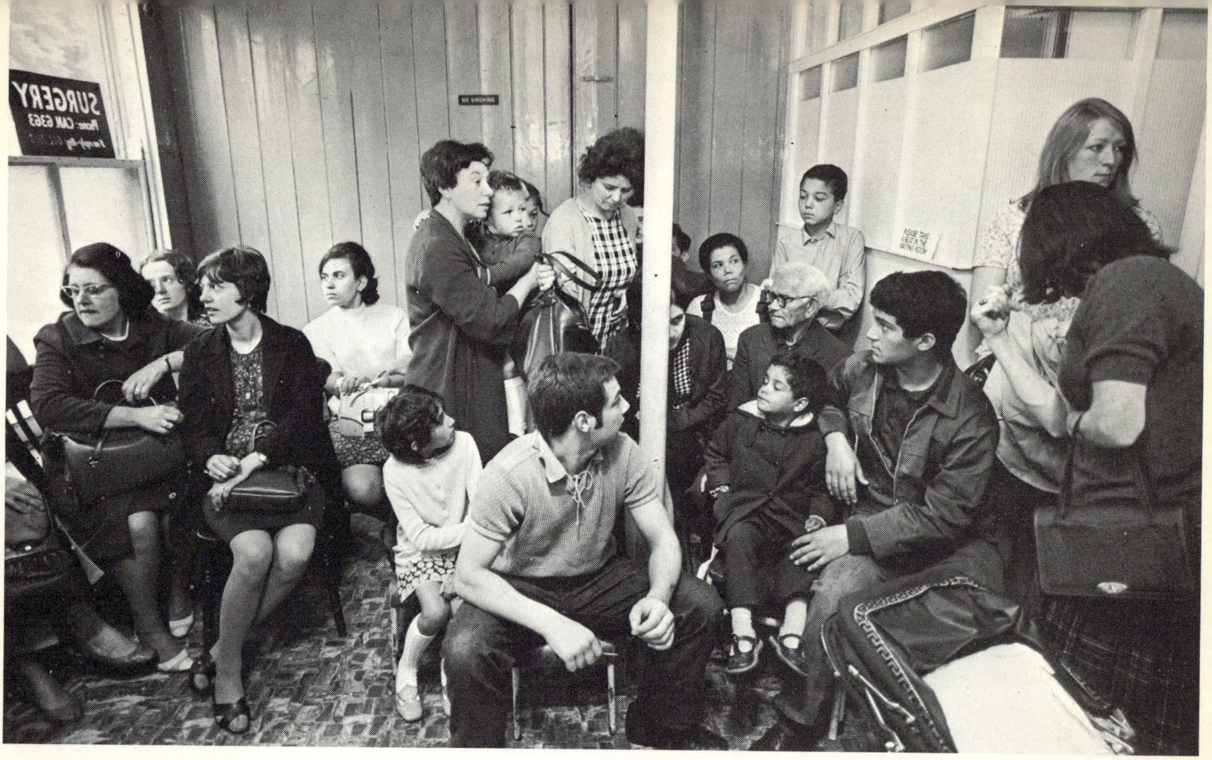

Even its greatest admirers would admit that the National Health Service has its shortcomings. Although it costs far more than anyone expected — at present about £1,500 million a year — it still suffers from a shortage of money. There are too few family doctors and many of them are overworked. Often, they have too little time to give to each patient, and seldom have the chance to catch up with the latest developments in medical science. Although the numbers of students at medical schools has been increased, it will be years before the benefits are felt. There are also too few hospitals and too few beds. A queue of 80,000 people, for example, waits to have their tonsils out; 76,000 people are in need of plastic surgery, while a seven-year wait for a simple operation like hernia or varicose veins is not unusual. Largely because of poor conditions or prospects, up to 900 doctors go abroad each year. Their place is taken by foreigners. Today nearly half the junior staff in all British hospitals were born outside the United Kingdom, and most of them in underdeveloped countries which need their services far more urgently than Britain does. Many of our 3,000

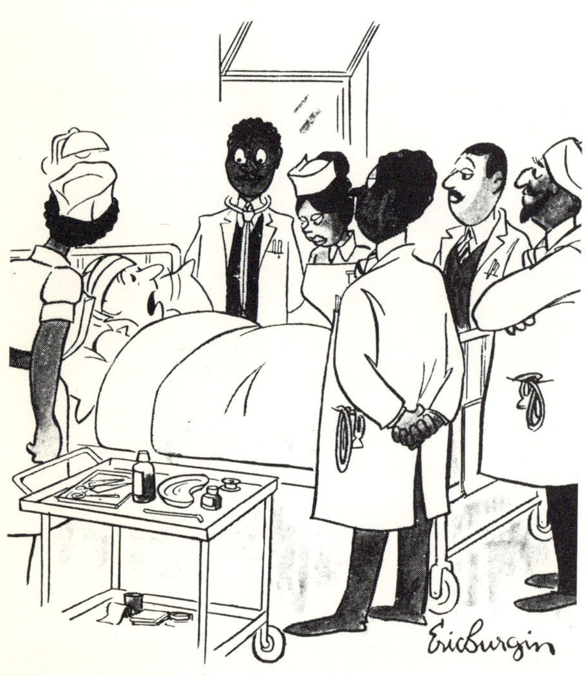

'Where am I?'

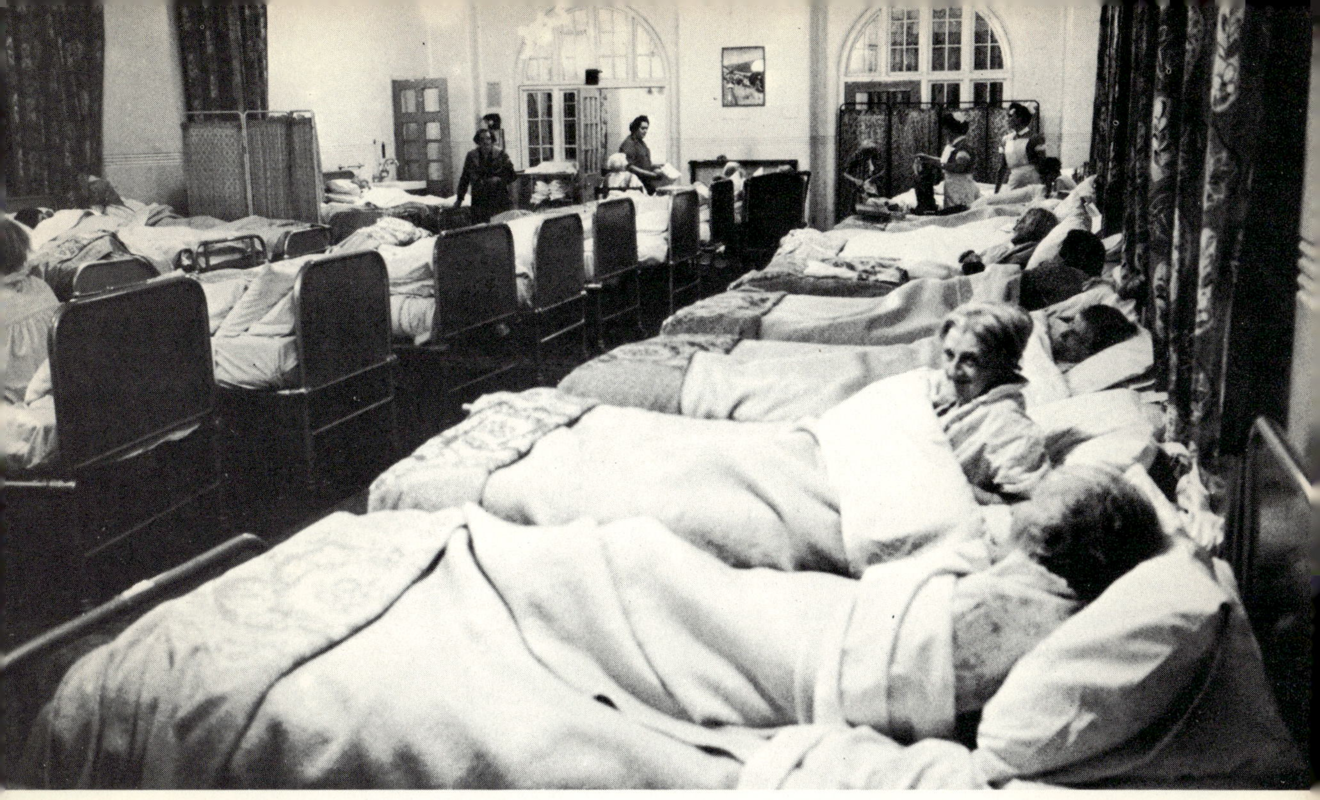

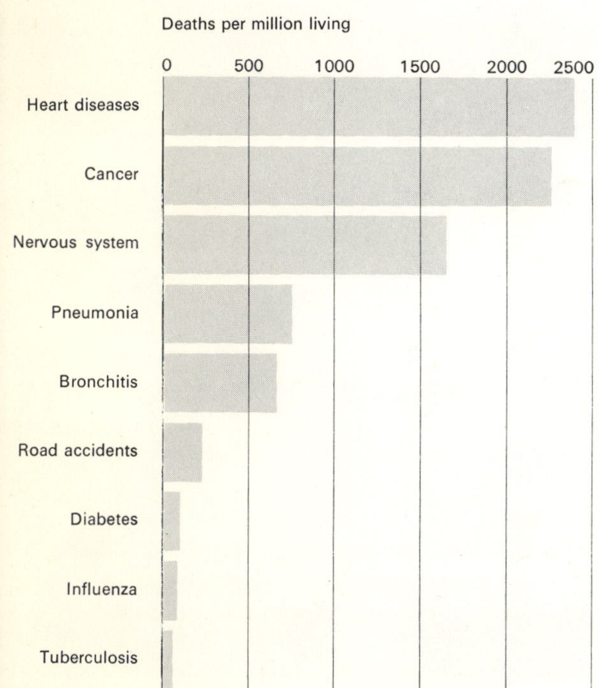

hospitals are out of date: one hospital in four is more than a century old, and only six new hospitals have been opened since 1939, too few even to keep pace with the rising population. Expensive modern equipment is often lacking: for example, there are only enough kidney machines to ensure treatment for 100 of the 20,000 people suffering from serious kidney disease. As a result of this more and more people are willing to pay extra for medical care by joining private insurance schemes which guarantee them immediate private treatment when ill. Already over a million people are covered by such schemes.

The diagram (left) shows the major causes of death in the United Kingdom between 1956 and 1966. The old epidemic diseases have completely vanished from the table, and only tuberculosis would probably appear on a similar list for the nineteenth century.

But modern society has created new problems and new causes of death. We eat well, we drive around in cars and trains, we take little exercise. Deaths from 'heart attacks', 'strokes', 'thrombosis' (clotting of the blood) are now the most serious cause of death, and often carry people off in early middle age.

We also have more money to spend on things like cigarettes, which we now know to be a major cause of lung cancer. Despite extensive research, doctors still do not know why certain cells in the body suddenly 'run wild' and begin to multiply until they form a malignant growth. Sometimes the doctor can check the growth, by surgery or radio-active exposure, and drugs may bring some relief to the patient. They *do* know, however, that cancer is a disease virtually unknown among native races living outdoors and eating natural foods.

Most of us, too, live in cities. Bronchitis, an inflammation of the tubes serving the lungs is far more common in the British Isles than anywhere else in the world, so that, as one doctor has written, 'this . . . might well be called the English disease'. After influenza, bronchitis is the most common cause of absence from work. The spread of smokeless zones may finally reverse the present trend, but it is unlikely that it will ever eliminate it.

There are still many problems which research has to solve. The most serious is probably cancer, but scientists are still baffled by an illness as ordinary and unserious as the common cold. Progress is slow, but study of an obscure disease affecting sheep has unexpectedly proved useful in solving the mystery of cancer. Similarly, a modern emphasis on research into viruses (very small germs which can only live inside living cells and not independently) has helped scientists to know a great deal more about the way the common cold virus works.

But the case of 'thalidomide children' stresses the dangers of trying to get quick results. Methods of testing new drugs and methods of treatment have greatly improved, though in this century there have been disasters in America with 'live' polio vaccine and in Australia with a diptheria anti-toxin. But the worst of all these accidents was thalidomide. Between 1960 and 1962 this drug was prescribed as a new form of sedative for pregnant women in several countries. The result was that many of their babies were born deformed. In Britain alone there are about 300 thalidomide children. There is no substitute for patience and exhaustive testing.

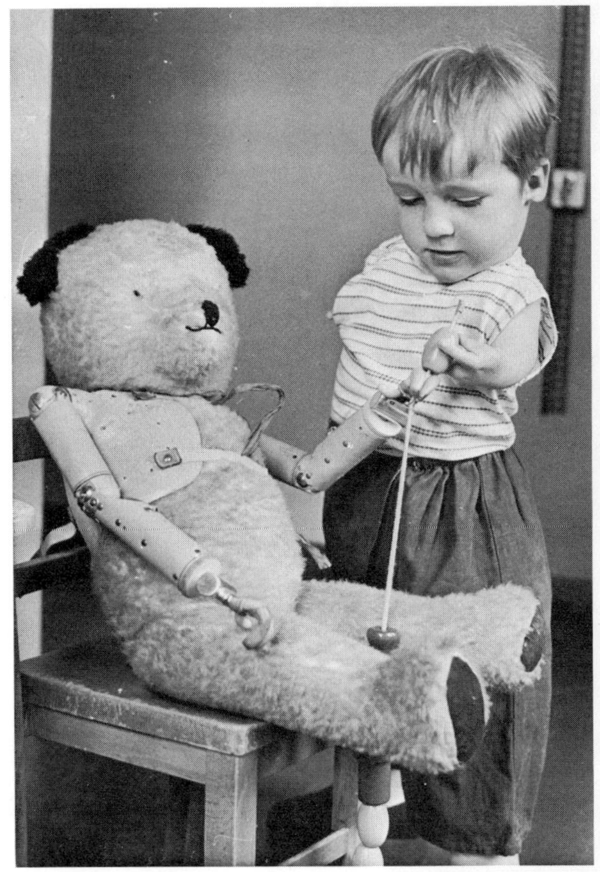

The future

In a now famous 'Brains Trust' programme on B.B.C. television in 1958 the 'most important scientific discovery in the next half-century' was discussed. The members of the panel were Professor A. J. Ayer (a philosopher), Professor W. Grey Walter (a neurologist), Aldous Huxley (novelist and writer), and Aldous Huxley's brother, Julian Huxley, an eminent biologist and writer. The panel agreed unanimously with Sir Julian: the most important scientific discovery would be the invention of an oral contraceptive. Oral contraceptives are now in use throughout the world. For the purposes of this book, we asked Sir Julian Huxley and two eminent scientists concerned with medical research to give their predictions about the future.

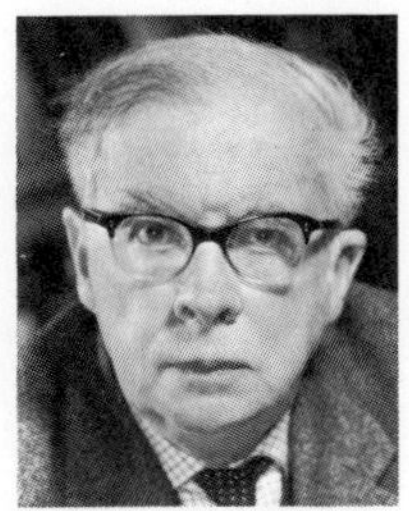

Sir Julian Huxley, F.R.S.

I am more than ever convinced that population increase is the most serious threat to civilization. It is becoming increasingly important to persuade people that they must limit their families, and that this can be done both by better contraceptive agents, like pills, *and* by increasing use of (reversible) sterilization of men. This last method is being increasingly used in India.

In medical research, we need to know more about the action of dangerous drugs like heroin, and how to prevent or cure addiction to them. And there is a need for more study of hallucinogenic substances like lysergic acid – L.S.D. – and their effects on consciousness. These effects are often very similar to those of mental diseases like schizophrenia, and a study of how to use hallucinogens for relief, while at the same time preventing their bad effects, will be very important. But the most fundamental medical discoveries will come in the field of cancer, its origin, prevention and cure.

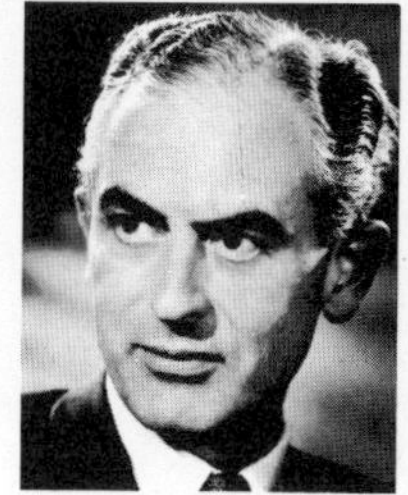

Professor Sir Peter Medawar, F.R.S.

Nobel Prizewinner in medicine and Director of the National Institute for Medical Research.

In my opinion the most important advance that can take place in medicine over the next twenty-five years is the extension to the world generally of the medical privileges at present enjoyed only by the advanced industrial countries. Beyond that, the next most important thing is to make further and more rapid progress with the elucidation of the organic causes of mental illnesses.

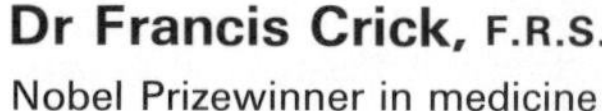

Dr Francis Crick, F.R.S.

Nobel Prizewinner in medicine

I am not medically qualified, but I suppose the most likely development in the near future will be advances in immunology, which will make the transplanting of organs much more successful than it is today. There does not seem much doubt that this will happen, but, of course, when it will happen is less certain.

As far as oral contraceptives are concerned, we may look forward to a 'male pill' and a 'morning-after pill'. However, if you were to ask me what effect medicine and public health is going to have on the next generation, I am afraid that one feature is likely to strike them more strongly than all the others put together. This is the tremendous increase in the percentage of senile people which is likely to take place over the next tens of years.

Further information

This list gives information about some books, places and things dealing with the history of public health and medicine.

Bibliography

Books more suitable for reference purposes because of their inclusiveness and length are marked □. Books suitable for younger readers are marked ■, but most of them are suitable for adults too. Most of the books published since 1950 are still in print. Earlier books should be available in large libraries, and some may be reprinted in any case by the time this book appears.

Source books

Most of these are very long, and written in old-fashioned styles, but they are invaluable because they contain detailed descriptions of the problems of public health as they seemed to people at the time.

□ Charles Booth, *Life and Labour of the People in London* (Macmillan, 1892–1903, 17 vols.). Indigestible if swallowed whole, but excellent in small pieces. Booth's immense and very detailed survey is concerned chiefly with poverty, but also includes many descriptions of the way in which the poor in London suffered from disease, bad housing and a defective public-health system.

□ Edwin Chadwick, *Report on the Sanitary Condition of the Labouring Population of Great Britain, 1842*, (Edinburgh University Press; new edition, 1965, with a long, very valuable, introductory essay by M. W. Flinn on the background to the report). Chadwick's report showed, in great detail and with vast intelligence, the link between dirt and disease. After its publication, the need for proper public-health measures could not be ignored by sensible people. It contains much graphic description of local conditions: look up your town in the index.

□ Henry Mayhew, *London Labour and the London Poor* (Frank Cass, 1967, 4 vols.). Mayhew's great book, first published in 1862, about the daily lives of the London poor in the 1850s contains much about the dirt and disease that they suffered from. In particular, in Volume 2 there is a long description of the streets and sewers of the city and how they were cleaned in the decade when modern sanitary engineering was just beginning. Also available is *Selections from London Labour and the London Poor*, ed. J. L. Bradley (Oxford University Press, 1965).

□ E. Royston Pike, *Human Documents of the Industrial Revolution in Britain* (Allen & Unwin paperback, 1966) and *Human Documents of the Victorian Golden Age* (Allen & Unwin, 1967). These two books contain short extracts from contemporary accounts of the lives of the poor: many deal with the public-health question. The Parliamentary Papers (sometimes called 'Blue Books') are the main sources. Pike gives full references which allows the reader easy access to this vast collection of material on Victorian social history.

Histories and biographies

Brian Abel-Smith, *A History of the Nursing Profession* (Heinemann, 1960) and *The Hospitals 1800–1948* (Heinemann, 1964). Two very scholarly and readable books with full bibliographies.

□ Maurice Bruce, *The Coming of the Welfare State* (Batsford, new edition, 1968). Places the public-health movement in the wide context of the development of state social provision since 1830. It is the best book available on this subject – detailed, thorough, interesting.

■ R. Calder, *From Magic to Medicine* (Macdonald, 1957). A lively and readable text with exceptionally good illustrations.
■ *The Story of Nursing* (Methuen 'Outlines' series, new edition, 1960). Deals with the history of nursing from Ancient Greece to the present day.

Hector Cameron, *Joseph Lister, Friend of Man* (Heinemann, 1948). A very readable account of Lister's life and work.

R. J. Cootes, *The Making of the Welfare State* (Longmans 'Modern Times' series, 1968). Twentieth-century developments – well written and illustrated.

■ P. Chambers, *Great Company: The Fight Against Disease* (Bodley Head, third edition, 1960). Short lives of the great medical pioneers – includes Semmelweiss and De Veuster as well as the more obvious ones.

■ J. G. Crowther, *Six Great Doctors* (Hamish Hamilton, 1957). Short lives of Fleming, Harvey, Lister, Pasteur, Pavlov and Ross.

□ Charles Creighton, *A History of Epidemics in Great Britain* originally published 1891–4, reprinted by Frank Cass, 1965. Two vast, rambling, detailed volumes. A rewarding quarry of unusual information, though the author's views on cholera are eccentric and misleading.

■ G. R. Davidson, *Medicine through the Ages* (Methuen 'Outlines' series, 1968).

G. Deaux, *The Black Death* (Hamish Hamilton, 1969). A well-written book about the great fourteenth-century pandemic.

■ E. Doorly, *Microbe Man* (Heinemann 'New Windmill' series, 1950). The classic life of Pasteur for younger readers. ■ *Radium Woman* 'New Windmill' series, 1949). A biography of Madame Curie. In some editions, both books are illustrated with fine woodcuts by Robert Gibbings.

R. and J. Dubos, *The White Plague* (Little, Brown, 1952). The standard book on the social history of tuberculosis and its cure. *Pasteur* (Little, Brown, 1950). A scholarly biography.

■ I. Eberle, *Edward Jenner and Smallpox Vaccination* (Chatto & Windus, 1963). A very good short account.

□ S. E. Finer, *The Life and Times of Sir Edwin Chadwick* (Methuen, 1952). One of the best books about Victorian social history. A detailed account of the early years of the public-health movement, though hard going for the reader.

M. W. Flinn, *Public Health Reform in Britain* (Macmillan, 1968). A short survey, devoted mainly to the nineteenth century. Well illustrated, scholarly and readable.

□ W. M. Frazer, *A History of English Public Health, 1834—1939* (Ballière, Tindall & Cassell, 1950). A straightforward and factual account.

A. H. Gale, *Epidemic Diseases* (Penguin Books, 1959). A short history of all the fatal diseases from the Middle Ages to the 1950s; not much about remedies.

R. J. Godlee, *Lister* (Macmillan, 1917). Still the best large biography of Lister.

■ E. Jenkins, *Joseph Lister* (Nelson, 1960). Good text, better illustrations.

□ Royston Lambert, *Sir John Simon, 1816—1904, and English Social Administration* (MacGibbon & Kee, 1963). The life of the great Victorian administrator of the State public-health service.

□ R. A. Lewis, *Edwin Chadwick and the Public Health Move-Ment, 1832—54* (Longmans, 1952). Very detailed.

Norman Longmate, *King Cholera* (Hamish Hamilton, 1966).

David Masters, *Miracle Drug: The Inner History of Penicillin* (Eyre & Spottiswood, 1946). A very readable account of the discovery of this vital drug.

André Maurois, *The life of Sir Alexander Fleming* (Cape, 1959; Penguin, 1963). A long, well-written and lively biography.

■ R. Mitchell, *A Country Doctor in the Reign of Queen Anne* (Longmans' 'Then and There' series, 1959). An excellent account of a doctor's life in an age of primitive medical science.

A. Newsholme, *Fifty Years in Public Health* (Allen & Unwin, 1935). An interesting autobiography of a medical officer of health.

Johannes Nohl, *The Black Death, A Chronicle of the Plague* (Allen & Unwin paperback, 1961). A short account containing many short extracts from contemporary writers.

■ N. Pain, *Louis Pasteur* (Black, 1957).

■ P. Pringle, *The Romance of Medical Science* (Harrap, 1948).

■ J. Rowland, *Chloroform Man: Dr James Simpson* (Lutterworth, 1961); ■ *Mosquito Man: Ronald Ross* (Lutterworth, 1958); ■ *Penicillin Man: Sir Alexander Fleming* (Lutterworth, 1957); ■ *Polio Man: Dr Salk* (Lutterworth, 1960). Four readable biographies.

□ John Simon, *English Sanitary Institutions* (Cassell, 1890). Still in many ways the best history of the public-health movement, by the man who was at the centre of it.

Cecil Woodham Smith, *Florence Nightingale* (Penguin Books, 1950). A readable though too uncritical biography of a great but, in her later years, remarkably narrow-minded woman.
■ *Lady in Chief* (Methuen, 1953) is an abridgement for young readers.

□ R. H. Shryock, *Development of Modern Medicine* (Knopf, 1947). Mainly concerned with the nineteenth century. His 'Medicine and Public Health', a long article in *The Nineteenth-Century World* (Mentor Books paperback, 1963) is an excellent survey of public-health movements and medical science in Europe (including Britain) and the United States in the last century. The only good survey of this general theme.

□ C. Singer and E. A. Underwood, *A Short History of Medicine* (Oxford University Press, second edition, 1959). Indispensable.

A. Swinson, *The Story of Public Health* (Pergamon, 1965). Informative.

■ J. Boswell Taylor, *Medicine* (Educational Supply Association, 1957). A good, brief survey. ■ *Edward Jenner: Conqueror of Smallpox* (Macmillan, 1950). A good biography, though perhaps too simple in places.

■ Roger Watson, *Edwin Chadwick: Poor Law and Public Health* (Longmans 'Then and There' series, 1969). The best short introduction to Chadwick's career and ideas for readers of any age. Contains much local material about public health in Darlington.

A. J. Willcocks, *The Creation of the National Health Service* (Routledge & Kegan Paul paperback, 1967). An intelligent account of the medieval pandemic: an excellent piece of socio- by the Labour party after the Second World War.

■ Norman Wymer, *Medical Scientists and Doctors* (Oxford University Press 'Lives of Great Men and Women' series, 1958). Imaginative and very readable biographies of Curie, Fleming, Harvey, Lister, Pasteur, Pavlov and Elizabeth Garrett Anderson, the first woman to be trained in England as a doctor. Each life is also available separately.

Philip Ziegler, *The Black Death* (Collins, 1969). The best account of the medieval pandemic: an excellent piece of socio-medical history.

Hans Zinsser, *Rats, Lice and History* (Bantam, 1965). As its title suggests, it deals with the pest-borne diseases — bubonic plague and typhus. Excellent.

Novels

Albert Camus, *The Plague* (Penguin Books, 1960). A sombre novel about the psychological effects of an epidemic of bubonic plague in a North African town in the twentieth century.

Daniel Defoe, *A Journal of the Plague Year* (Penguin Books, 1966). A novel about the last great outbreak of bubonic plague in Britain — the London plague of 1665. Not, strictly speaking, a contemporary account, since Defoe was only five years old in 1665 and of course wrote his book many years later. It is based, however, on conversations he had with people who lived through the plague.

Benjamin Disraeli, *Sybil: or the Two Nations* (Nelson, 1950). First published in 1845. A mannered, ironic and often irritating novel — one of the first to introduce the public-health question into fiction. Contains description of the dirt and disease in 'Wodgate', an imaginary Northern industrial town.

Charles Kingsley, *Alton Locke, Tailor and Poet* (Cassell, 1967). First published 1850. Very hard reading today: but Chapter 35 contains a brilliant description of the conditions in Bermondsey which helped to cause epidemics of cholera. *Two Years Ago*. First published 1856, now out of print. Quite hard to read, but contains an interesting account of a cholera epidemic in a seaside village in Cornwall.

Sinclair Lewis, *Arrowsmith* (Signet, 1967). First published 1924. Excellent novel about medical research and doctors' attempts to deal with the plague on the imaginary West Indian island of St Hubert.

Local sources

As the first chapter of this book shows, public health was a far greater problem in urban than in rural areas. By our standards, the latter were insanitary in the 1840s: indeed many of them still are today, however picturesque. But being relatively small then, the problem could be ignored, and usually was. Thus rural public health has no history, or at least none that can be investigated easily without delving into a mass of obscure archive material. In towns, however, the recognition of the problem produced a vast quantity of print in the 1840s and 50s, much of it accessible today. Chadwick's *Report* contains a great deal of information about specific towns and cities; Flinn's introduction and Royston Pike's books give references to other Parliamentary Papers that contain similar material. These references only skim the possibilities: the list of appropriate Parliamentary Papers is vast. An invaluable general guide is W. R. Powell, *Local History from Blue Books*, an Historical Association pamphlet published in 1962.

One advantage of the Parliamentary Papers is that you can get useful material from them *quickly*. Most university libraries, and many civic libraries (e.g. Manchester and Birmingham) have good runs of them. They are copiously indexed and evidence relating to each town is often printed coherently and can be xeroxed cheaply. Much other local material which yields quick results may also be found in local libraries and record offices. Common, and very useful, are the reports that the local inspectors of the General Board of Health made in the 1840s and 50s on the sanitary state of individual towns, and the spate of pamphlets produced by interested parties on the public-health question locally. It is a lengthy and laborious task to work continuously through local newspapers, but it is often worth scanning short runs for specific dates — for example, the last three months of 1831 (cholera), the last six months of 1848 (the public-health question) or the last two months of 1918 (the 'Spanish flu' epidemic). One excellent book that draws upon some of this local material for Darlington is Roger Watson, *Edwin Chadwick, Poor Law and Public Health.*

The standard modern histories of towns often contain much about public health. In addition, there are a few books on local history devoted to the question:

A. K. Chalmers, *The Health of Glasgow, 1818–1925* (Glasgow Corporation, 1930).

James Niven, *History of Public Health Effort in Manchester* (1923).

W. M. Frazer, *Duncan of Liverpool* (Hamish Hamilton, 1947). The biography of the first municipal medical officer of health.

Museums

Some medical schools have museums for their students but members of the general public are not admitted. Listed here are several museums which have medical and public-health collections and which are open to the public. By far the most important is:

The Wellcome Institute of the History of Medicine, Euston Road, London NW1; open Monday–Friday, 10–5; Saturday, 9.30–4.30. The largest collections of medical and public-health material in the world, ranging from prehistoric times to the present day.

Also:

Edinburgh: *Museum of Childhood*, 34 High Street; open weekdays, 10–5. Includes material on the health of children.

Edinburgh: *Museum of the Royal College of Surgeons of Edinburgh*, may be opened for visitors, by appointment.

Liverpool: *Museum of the School of Hygiene*, 126 Mount Pleasant; open Monday–Friday, 9–4.30. Collection of public-health exhibits 'mainly of interest to students'.

London: *The Health Exhibition Centre*, 90 Buckingham Palace Road, SW1; open Monday–Friday, 10–5. Permanent exhibition of modern public-health topics.

London: *Pharmaceutical Society's Museum*, 17 Bloomsbury Square, WC1; open by arrangement. Exhibitions of drugs and chemists' equipment.

London: *Royal College of Surgeons' Museum*, Lincolns Inn Fields, WC2. Exhibitions of surgical equipment; open by arrangement.

Oxford: *Museum of the History of Science*, Broad Street; open weekdays, 10.30–1, 2.30–4. Includes a few exhibits dealing with medical and pharmaceutical history

Winslow, Buckinghamshire: *Florence Nightingale Museum*, Claydon House, which belongs to the National Trust; open March–October, Tuesday–Sunday, 2–6. Large collection relating to Florence Nightingale and her nursing activities.

Visual material

There are 'Jackdaws' (Jonathan Cape) on *The Plague and the Fire of London, The Black Death* and *The Crimean War*. There is also a 'Science Jackdaw' on *Pasteur and the Germ Theory* (good, but sometimes hard going for non-scientists).

Several of the museums publish postcards and slides.

A film, 'The Story of Penicillin', may be borrowed free from I.C.I. Filmstrips are produced by Common Ground (44 Fulham Road, London SW3) on 'The Curies and Radium', 'Lister and Antiseptics', 'Pasteur and Microbes'; and by Hulton Educational Productions (55–9 Saffron Hill, London EC1) on 'The History of Medicine'.

Magazine

World Health, an illustrated magazine published every two months by the World Health Organization, Division of Public Information, Palais des Nations, Geneva, Switzerland (copies can be bought in the United Kingdom from branches of H.M. Stationery Office).

Index

Numbers in italics refer to the captions of illustrations and maps.

Acknowledgements

The author and publishers would like to thank many people for their help in preparing this book. Sir Julian Huxley, Professor Sir Peter Medawar and Dr Francis Crick responded very readily to our request for their views on the future. Mr E. Gaskell, Librarian of the Wellcome Institute of the History of Medicine, gave us a great deal of detailed help with the charts. Dr Ian MacQueen, in 1964, as now, Medical Officer of Health for the City of Aberdeen, very kindly checked the 'Diary of an Epidemic'. Peter Searby's interest and advice have been invaluable at all stages, and he also prepared the section of 'Further Information'. Dr Grace Adam also gave some helpful advice.

The author acknowledges with thanks the assistance of Mrs Sue Sabbagh, who did some of the research; of Mrs Sheila Bailey, who prepared the manuscript; and of Dr Florence Cadogan of the Greater London Public Health Service, who kindly read through it and offered advice at every stage.

Illustration acknowledgements

page

7–8 Mansell Collection
9 Punch Publications Ltd
10 Mansell Collection
12 Punch Publications Ltd
13 From the *London Graphic*, 1876
14 Radio Times Hulton Picture Library
15 From the *Comic Almanack*, 1845
16 Mansell Collection
17 Wellcome Historical Medical Museum and Library/from *New Inventions* by Maurice Richards, published by Hugh Evelyn Ltd
18 Punch Publications Ltd
19 Wellcome Historical Medical Museum and Library/ Victoria and Albert Museum
23–5 Sunderland Public Libraries, Museum and Art Gallery
27 British Museum/Welcome Historical Medical Museum and Library
28 Dudley Public Libraries/Bilston Public Library
29 Bilston Public Library
31 Radio Times Hulton Picture Library
33 Wellcome Historical Medical Museum and Library
34 Wellcome Historical Medical Museum and Library/ Radio Times Hulton Picture Library
36 Wellcome Historical Medical Museum and Library/ Mansell Collection
37 Mansell Collection/Wellcome Historical Medical Museum and Library
39 Wellcome Historical and Medical Museum and Library
40 Radio Times Hulton Picture Library
42 Wellcome Historical and Medical Museum and Library
43 Punch Publications Ltd
44 Mansell Collection
45 Wellcome Historical Medical Museum and Library
47 Metropolitan Water Board
48 Mansell Collection
49 Wellcome Historical Medical Museum and Library
52 Wellcome Historical Medical Museum and Library
53 Punch Publications Ltd
54 Aldus Books/Mansell Collection
55 Wellcome Historical Medical Museum and Library
57 Photograph Keith Morris
59–60 Wellcome Historical Medical Museum and Library
61 The President and Council, The Royal College of Surgeons of England
64 Mansell Collection
67 Wellcome Historical Medical Museum and Library
68 Mansell Collection
69 Mansell Collection/Keystone Press Agency Ltd
70 The Bettmann Archive Inc./The Trustees, Hammersmith Hospital
71 Radio Times Hulton Picture Library/North-West Metropolitan Regional Hospital Board
73 Wellcome Historical Medical Museum and Library/Radio Times Hulton Picture Library
74 The Wellcome Historical Medical Museum and Library/ Mansell Collection
75 Mansell Collection/Musée de l'Institut Pasteur
76 Radio Times Hulton Picture Library
77 Health Education Council, Department of Health and Social Security and Central Office of Information
78 Radio Times Hulton Picture Library
80 St Mary's Hospital Medical School
81 Glaxo Laboratories Ltd
84 The Bodley Head
86 Radio Times Hulton Picture Library
87 Frank Staff
88 Radio Times Hulton Picture Library
89 Punch Publications Ltd
90 Radio Times Hulton Picture Library
93 Thomson Newspapers Ltd
94 Photographs Geoffrey Drury
95 Aerofilms
96 Photograph John Brooke/Punch Publications Ltd
97 Photograph John Brooke
98 Camera Press Ltd
99 Paul Popper Ltd / Photograph Godfrey Argent / Camera Press Ltd